Osteoporosis

Guest Editor

STUART L. SILVERMAN, MD

RHEUMATIC DISEASE CLINICS OF NORTH AMERICA

www.rheumatic.theclinics.com

August 2011 • Volume 37 • Number 3

SAUNDERS an imprint of ELSEVIER, Inc.

W.B. SAUNDERS COMPANY

A Division of Elsevier Inc.

1600 John F. Kennedy Blvd., Suite 1800 • Philadelphia, PA 19103-2899

http://www.theclinics.com

RHEUMATIC DISEASE CLINICS OF NORTH AMERICA Volume 37, Number 3

August 2011 ISSN 0889-857X, ISBN 13: 978-1-4557-7991-8

Editor: Rachel Glover

Rheumatic Disease Clinics of North America (ISSN 0889-857X) is published quarterly by Elsevier Inc., 360 Park Avenue South, New York, NY 10010-1710. Months of issue are February, May, August, and November. Business and editorial offices: 1600 John F. Kennedy Boulevard, Suite 1800, Philadelphia, PA 19103-2899. Periodicals postage paid at New York, NY and additional mailing offices. Subscription prices are USD 282.00 per year for US individuals, USD 501.00 per year for US institutions, USD 139.00 per year for US students and residents, USD 333.00 per year for Canadian individuals, USD 619.00 per year for Canadian institutions, USD 395.00 per year for international individuals, USD 619.00 per year for international institutions, and USD 194.00 per year for Canadian and foreign students/residents. To receive student/resident rate, orders must be accompanied by name of affiliated institution, date of term, and the *signature* of program/residency coordinator on institution letterhead. Orders will be billed at individual rate until proof of status received. Foreign air speed delivery is included in all *Clinics* subscription prices. All prices are subject to change without notice. **POSTMASTER:** Send address changes to *Rheumatic Disease Clinics of North America,* Elsevier Health Sciences Division, Subscription Customer Service, 3251 Riverport Lane, Maryland Heights, MO 63043. **Customer Service: 1-800-654-2452 (US and Canada). From outside of the US and Canada: 314-447-8871. Fax: 314-447-8029. For print support, e-mail: JournalsCustomerService-usa@elsevier.com. For online support, e-mail: JournalsOnline Support-usa@elsevier.com.**

Reprints. For copies of 100 or more of articles in this publication, please contact the Commercial Reprints Department, Elsevier Inc., 360 Park Avenue South, New York, New York, 10010-1710; Tel.: (+1) 212-633-3813, Fax: (+1) 212-462-1935, and E-mail: reprints@elsevier.com.

Rheumatic Disease Clinics of North America is covered in *MEDLINE/PubMed (Index Medicus), Current Contents/Clinical Medicine, Science Citation Index, ISI/BIOMED,* and *EMBASE/Excerpta Medica.*

Printed and bound by CPI Group (UK) Ltd, Croydon, CR0 4YY

Transferred to Digital Print 2011

Contributors

GUEST EDITOR

STUART L. SILVERMAN, MD, FACP, FACR
Medical Director, Cedars-Sinai Bone Center of Excellence; Clinical Professor of Medicine,
University of California Los Angeles, Los Angeles; Medical Director, OMC Clinical
Research Center, Beverly Hills, California

AUTHORS

SANFORD BAIM, MD
Associate Professor of Clinical Medicine, Division of Endocrinology, Miller School
of Medicine, University of Miami, Miami, Florida

YVES BOUTSEN, MD
Division of Rheumatology and Rheumatology Unit, Université Catholique de Louvain,
Saint-Luc University Hospital, Brussels; Professor of Rheumatology, Division of
Rheumatology, Department of Medicine, University Hospital in Mont-Godinne,
Yvoir, Belgium

NANCY CHILES, BS
Department of Epidemiology and Public Health, School of Medicine, University
of Maryland; Doctoral Candidate, Doctoral Program in Gerontology, School of Medicine,
University of Maryland, Baltimore, Maryland

JEFFREY R. CURTIS, MD, MS, MPH
Division of Clinical Immunology and Rheumatology, University of Alabama at Birmingham,
Birmingham, Alabama

CHAD DEAL, MD
Staff Physician Cleveland Clinic, Associate Professor of Medicine, Head, Department
of Rheumatology, Center for Osteoporosis and Metabolic Bone Disease, Cleveland Clinic
Lerner College of Medicine at Case Western Reserve University, Cleveland Clinic,
Cleveland, Ohio

JEAN-PIERRE DEVOGELAER, MD
Professor Emeritus of Rheumatology, Division of Rheumatology and Rheumatology Unit,
Department of Medicine, Université Catholique de Louvain, Saint-Luc University Hospital,
Brussels, Belgium

ROBIN K. DORE, MD
Clinical Professor of Medicine, Division of Rheumatology, David Geffen School
of Medicine, University of California, Los Angeles, California

DAMIEN GRUSON, CP
Clinical Pathologist, Department of Laboratory Medicine; Department of Clinical
Biochemistry and the Rheumatology Unit, Université Catholique de Louvain, Saint-Luc
University Hospital, Brussels, Belgium

MARC C. HOCHBERG, MD, MPH
Professor of Medicine and Epidemiology and Public Health, Department of Medicine,
School of Medicine, University of Maryland, Baltimore, Maryland

MARK JONES, BS
Department of Epidemiology and Public Health, School of Medicine, University
of Maryland; Doctoral Candidate, Epidemiology Doctoral Program, School of Medicine,
University of Maryland, Baltimore, Maryland

ANDREW J. LASTER, MD
Private Practice, Arthritis and Osteoporosis Consultants of the Carolinas, Charlotte,
North Carolina

DANIEL MANICOURT, MD, PhD
Professor of Rheumatology, Division of Rheumatology and Rheumatology Unit,
Department of Medicine, Université Catholique de Louvain, Saint-Luc University Hospital,
Brussels, Belgium

MICHAEL MARICIC, MD
Associate Professor of Clinical Medicine, University of Arizona School of Medicine;
Catalina Pointe Rheumatology, Tucson, Arizona

KEATON NASSER, MD, FACP, FACR
Researcher, OMC Clinical Research Center, Beverly Hills, California

DENISE L. ORWIG, PhD
Department of Epidemiology and Public Health, School of Medicine, University
of Maryland, Baltimore, Maryland

KENNETH G. SAAG, MD, MSc
Division of Clinical Immunology and Rheumatology, University of Alabama at Birmingham,
Birmingham, Alabama

DAVID S. SILVER, MD
Cedars-Sinai Medical Center; University of Los Angeles School of Medicine, Los Angeles;
OMC Clinical Research Center, Beverly Hills, California

STUART L. SILVERMAN, MD, FACP, FACR
Medical Director, Cedars-Sinai Bone Center of Excellence; Clinical Professor of Medicine,
University of California Los Angeles, Los Angeles; Medical Director, OMC Clinical
Research Center, Beverly Hills, California

S. BOBO TANNER, MD
Divisions of Rheumatology and Allergy and Immunology, Vanderbilt University Medical
Center, Nashville, Tennessee

JIE ZHANG, PhD
Health Services/Comparative Effectiveness Research Training Program, Department
of Epidemiology, University of Alabama at Birmingham, Birmingham, Alabama

Contents

Preface: Osteoporosis   ix

Stuart L. Silverman

Duration of Treatment in Postmenopausal Osteoporosis: How Long to Treat and What are the Consequences of Cessation of Treatment?   323

Andrew J. Laster and S. Bobo Tanner

Although a variety of medications are effective for the treatment of postmenopausal osteoporosis, there is concern that long-term use may incur side effects. Consequently, some have proposed discontinuing or temporarily suspending treatment after a defined period of time. As the benefits of fracture risk reduction may recede during this "drug holiday", the clinician may be faced with deciding when to resume therapy (and with which agent) while avoiding the possible cumulative risk of side effects. This article summarizes data regarding length of treatment and the effects of cessation of treatment on bone density, bone turnover markers, and fracture risk.

Emerging Therapies for Osteoporosis   337

Chad Deal

This article reviews the conceptual framework for agents that are antiresorptive or anabolic, including pathways that affect bone formation and resorption, and the steps in those pathways that are targets for new therapeutic agents. This article discusses novel antiresorptive and anabolic agents in development. Recent developments that link bone remodeling with serotonin in the gastrointestinal system and the central nervous system via the sympathetic nervous system may change the paradigm for skeletal remodeling. Novel anabolic agents in development include antibodies that target molecules involved in Wnt signaling.

Calcium and Vitamin D Controversies   351

David S. Silver

Controversies regarding appropriate use of vitamin D and calcium are predominately related to the extraskeletal effects. Calcium and vitamin D are essential for bone health. The concerns regarding calcium and cardiovascular complications are inconclusive at best, and do not warrant a change in our approach to supplementation at this time. A growing body of literature exists suggesting that additional vitamin D may have numerous benefits, although more study needs to be done. Further prospective trials would provide insight into the potential advantages that increased vitamin D supplementation could provide.

Is There a Place for Bone Turnover Markers in the Assessment of Osteoporosis and its Treatment?   365

Jean-Pierre Devogelaer, Yves Boutsen, Damien Gruson, and Daniel Manicourt

As populations age, the number of osteoporotic fractures will increase. Bone mineral density (BMD) measurement remains the major way to diagnose osteoporosis and to indicate therapy. The FRAX tool, based on clinical risk factors, estimates the 10-year risk of hip and major osteoporotic fractures. The association of BMD and FRAX measurements has improved the identification of patients who are most at risk. However, some patients can still be overlooked and denied therapy. It is sound that adding the measure of bone turnover markers to the former risk factors and their follow-up during therapy could best address the efficacy of treatment of osteoporosis. Whether this behavior is cost-effective remains to be settled.

Long-term Safety Concerns of Antiresorptive Therapy   387

Jie Zhang, Kenneth G. Saag, and Jeffrey R. Curtis

Bisphosphonates reduce the risk of major osteoporotic fractures and are the most commonly used medications for the prevention and treatment of osteoporosis. Although these medications are well tolerated and safe during large-scale clinical trials, several rare and serious adverse events are suspected to be associated with long-term bisphosphonate use. These adverse events include osteonecrosis of the jaw, atypical fractures, and esophageal cancer. This review summarizes studies examining the association between bisphosphonate use and these adverse outcomes, with a focus on large case series and controlled epidemiologic studies.

Osteoporosis in Men: Update 2011   401

Denise L. Orwig, Nancy Chiles, Mark Jones, and Marc C. Hochberg

During the past year several review articles have been published on the topic of osteoporosis in men. These reviews have highlighted recommendations for measuring bone mineral density (BMD) in older men as a means of screening for osteoporosis, use of the World Health Organization's Fracture Risk Assessment Tool for predicting the risk of hip and major osteoporotic fractures, frequency of secondary causes of osteoporosis, useful laboratory tests to evaluate these conditions, newer treatments for men with osteoporosis that increase BMD and may reduce the risk of fractures, and new data on the prevalence of low BMD and osteoporosis in men.

Update on Glucocorticoid-Induced Osteoporosis   415

Michael Maricic

Glucocorticoid-induced osteoporosis (GIOP) is the most common form of secondary osteoporosis, and fractures are the most frequent adverse effects of this medication. Glucocorticoids have several direct and indirect adverse effects on bone, primarily through reduction in osteoblasts and osteocyte activity, and life span. Recent advances in the pathophysiology and prevention of this complication of therapy provide hope for its amelioration in patients being treated with glucocorticoids. Several effective pharmacologic agents are now available, and guidelines for the prevention and treatment of GIOP have been published. Despite these advances, many patients still do not receive proper prevention or therapy.

The RANKL Pathway and Denosumab   433

Robin K. Dore

Denosumab (Prolia) is a fully human monoclonal antibody directed against receptor activator of nuclear factor-κB ligand (RANKL), which interferes with the formation, activation, and survival of osteoclasts. It was approved by the Food and Drug Administration in June 2010 as a new treatment for postmenopausal osteoporosis in women who are at high risk for fracture. Given its mechanism of action, it is an antiresorptive therapy that is administered as a 60-mg subcutaneous injection every 6 months. It is the first biologic antiresorptive therapy for osteoporosis, and the first osteoporosis therapy to show efficacy and safety in patients with renal impairment.

Assessment of Fracture Risk 453

Sanford Baim

Osteoporosis-related fractures are associated with significant morbidity, mortality, and health care expenditure worldwide. The low sensitivity of bone density testing alone to predict fractures has led to the development of a variety of fracture assessment tools that use the combination of bone density and clinical risk factors to improve the prediction of low-trauma fractures. These fracture assessment tools quantitatively predict the 10-year probability of hip and major osteoporosis-related fractures, and can be used with various intervention strategies to effectively intervene with cost-effective therapies to prevent future fractures.

Teriparitide Update 471

Stuart L. Silverman and Keaton Nasser

Teriparitide (TPD) is a novel anabolic agent that stimulates bone formation. TPD reduces risk of vertebral and nonvertebral fracture. Due to its positive effects on bone formation, many new uses of TPD are being explored. It has been studied and approved for glucocorticoid-induced osteoporosis. Many questions about the use of TPD remain including use of follow-up therapy, combination therapy, sequential therapy, and its potential role in fracture healing and treatment of back pain related to osteoporosis.

Index 479

FORTHCOMING ISSUES

November 2011
Rheumatic Manifestations of Cancer
Charles R. Thomas Jr, MD, and
Kenneth Scalapino, MD,
Guest Editors

February 2012
Early Arthritis
Karina Torralba, MD, and
Richard S. Panush, MD,
Guest Editors

RECENT ISSUES

May 2011
Myopathies
Robert L. Wortmann, MD, *Guest Editor*

February 2011
**Complementary and Alternative Medicine
in Rheumatology**
Sharon L. Kolasinski, MD, *Guest Editor*

November 2010
**Rheumatologic Manifestations
of Endocrine Disease**
Joseph A. Markenson, MD,
Guest Editor

RELATED INTEREST

Endocrinology and Metabolism Clinics of North America, Volume 39,
Issue 2 (June 2010)
Vitamin D
Sol Epstein, MD, *Guest Editor*

THE CLINICS ARE NOW AVAILABLE ONLINE!

Access your subscription at:
www.theclinics.com

Preface

Osteoporosis

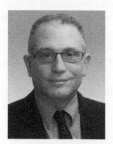

Stuart L. Silverman, MD
Guest Editor

This issue of *Rheumatic Disease Clinics of North America* is dedicated to the efforts of rheumatologists worldwide to study, diagnose, and treat osteoporosis. Rheumatologists are uniquely positioned to treat osteoporosis as patients with osteoporosis often present with the painful symptoms of fracture. Rheumatologists treat patients with diseases associated with increased risk of fracture such as rheumatoid arthritis or use medications like glucocorticoids, which increase the risk of fracture. Rheumatologists are often the champions for osteoporosis in their own institutions and local communities.

Rheumatologists have taken the lead in many aspects of the osteoporosis world globally, nationally, and locally. Rheumatologists have led national organizations such as International Society of Clinical Densitometry (ISCD) and American Society for Bone Mineral Research (ASBMR).

The American College of Rheumatology or ACR has had a study group in osteoporosis metabolic bone disease for almost two decades. The ACR has taken the lead in developing guidelines for glucocorticoid-induced osteoporosis.

Rheumatologists have participated in ASBMR taskforces on system-wide intervention, osteonecrosis of the jaw, and atypical fractures.

Rheumatologists have participated in developing new accreditation criteria for osteoporosis for the Joint Commission.

Rheumatologists have taken the lead studying the health-related quality-of-life impact of osteoporosis.

In this issue, we invited rheumatology osteoporosis experts and their colleagues to discuss the ten following topics related to the assessment and treatment of osteoporosis.

1. Sandy Baim from the University of Miami updates us on the strengths and limitation of FRAX, the new WHO fracture risk algorithm, which helps us to target the patients who need treatment the most.
2. David Silver from Cedars-Sinai tries to make sense of the current calcium and vitamin D controversy.

Rheum Dis Clin N Am 37 (2011) ix–x
doi:10.1016/j.rdc.2011.08.003
0889-857X/11/$ – see front matter © 2011 Elsevier Inc. All rights reserved.

3. Jie Zhang, Ken Saag, and Jeff Curtis from the University of Alabama at Birmingham address the adverse effects associated with long-term bisphosphonate therapy and discuss osteonecrosis of the jaw and atypical fractures.
4. Andy Laster from Arthritis and Osteoporosis Consultants of the Carolinas, and Bobo Tanner from Vanderbilt University have cogently reviewed the issues of discontinuing long-term bisphosphonate therapy and possibly taking a holiday. We can no longer treat patients with risk for fracture with a single drug during their lifetime.
5. Robin Dore from UCLA shares with us new data of up to 5 years on denosumab, the first RANK-ligand inhibitor.
6. Mike Maricic from the University of Arizona updates us on glucocorticoid osteoporosis, both the identification of patients who should be treated by ACR criteria as well as the new management options.
7. As we begin to place our bisphosphonate patients on holidays, the importance of being able to monitor patients has increased. J.P. Devogelaer, Yves Boutsen, Damein Gruson, and Daniel Manicourt from the Université Catholique de Louvain give us some guidelines on the place of bone turnover markers in osteoporosis assessment and treatment.
8. Denise Orwig, Nancy Chiles, Mark Jones, and Marc Hochberg from the University of Maryland update us on the treatment of osteoporosis in men.
9. Chad Deal from the Cleveland Clinic discusses exciting data on new osteoporosis drugs, particularly the new anabolics.
10. Finally, with my colleague Keaton Nasser from Cedars-Sinai, I discuss an update on teriparatide, the first approved anabolic therapy.

Enjoy!

Stuart L. Silverman, MD
Cedars-Sinai Bone Center of Excellence
8641 Wilshire Boulevard, Suite 301
Los Angeles, CA 90211, USA

E-mail address:
stuarts@omcresearch.org

Duration of Treatment in Postmenopausal Osteoporosis: How Long to Treat and What are the Consequences of Cessation of Treatment?

Andrew J. Laster, MD[a],*, S. Bobo Tanner, MD[b,c]

KEYWORDS

• Osteoporosis • Drug holiday • Fracture risk • Bisphosphonate
• Teriparatide • Raloxifene • Denosumab • Estrogen

There are few concerns about the consequences of long-term treatment of chronic disease except when the drugs being used accumulate within the body. Rheumatologists are well aware of the affinity of the choloroquines for the retina and its resulting ocular toxicity in select individuals. Bisphosphonates avidly bind to hydroxyapatite within bone and have limited biological degradation.[1–3] Although causality has not been definitively established, concern that bisphosphonate therapy could lead to specific bone toxicities such as osteonecrosis of the jaw (ONJ), and atypical fractures can be appreciated in this construct. Whether other potent antiresorptives such as denosumab, which do not bind to bone, have similar toxicities remains unanswered at this time.

In addition, there has been an appreciation that patients who have been treated with select bisphosphonates for several years could stop taking the drug without a rapid

Financial Disclosure/Conflict of Interest: A.J.L.: Consulting/Speakers Bureau: Amgen, Genentech, Lilly, Novartis, Roche GSK. S.B.T.: Consulting/Honoraria/Research Support: Amgen, Pfizer, Lilly, Merck, Novartis, Genentech, Roche, UCB, Centocor, AstraZeneca, BMS.
[a] Arthritis & Osteoporosis Consultants of the Carolinas, 1918 Randolph Road, Suite 600, Charlotte, NC 28207, USA
[b] Division of Rheumatology, Vanderbilt University Medical Center, 2611 West End Avenue, Suite 210, Nashville, TN 37203, USA
[c] Division of Allergy & Immunology, Vanderbilt University Medical Center, Nashville, TN, USA
* Corresponding author.
E-mail address: ajlaster@aocc.md

Rheum Dis Clin N Am 37 (2011) 323–336
doi:10.1016/j.rdc.2011.07.007
0889-857X/11/$ – see front matter © 2011 Elsevier Inc. All rights reserved.

rheumatic.theclinics.com

decline in bone density or increase in markers of bone resorption. Some have taken this residual effect on bone density and bone turnover markers to imply continued fracture benefit even after drug cessation. However, studies demonstrating persistent fracture benefit are limited.

This review examines the different drug therapies currently approved by the Food and Drug Administration (FDA) for use in the management of postmenopausal osteoporosis, and evaluates the current data regarding effects of discontinuation on bone mineral density (BMD), bone turnover markers (BTM), and fracture risk reduction. The authors attempt to provide a general framework for clinicians to determine which patients are appropriate candidates for discontinuation of medical therapy, temporary suspension (drug holiday), and continued treatment. Two other excellent reviews on this topic with somewhat contrasting recommendations have appeared within the last 2 years, by Seeman[4] and Watts and Diab.[5]

There are other questions implicit in this discussion. What is the optimal duration of treatment with these agents in achieving fracture reduction and avoiding side effects related to cumulative exposure? What effect does a "holiday" have on the reduction of the risk of side effects? Does resumption of treatment after a holiday resume the risk? Does a change from an antiresorptive agent to an anabolic agent reset the cumulative risk of the antiresorptive agent back to baseline? Does a change in the mechanism of antiresorptive treatment (eg, bisphosphonate versus denosumab) change the cumulative risk? Unfortunately, there are currently few data to guide the answers to these important questions, yet clinicians are faced with these decisions daily.

DISCONTINUING OSTEOPOROSIS TREATMENT
The Effect on Bone Mineral Density and Bone Turnover Markers

Cessation of osteoporosis treatment has been shown to have a range of effects on BMD as well as BTM.

Bisphosphonates

Clinical trials demonstrate significant differences in the bisphosphonates regarding BMD and BTM following discontinuation of therapy. The effect of 1 year (1 dose) of zolendronate appears to persist for at least 3 years in women with osteopenia.[6] In patients with osteoporosis, alendronate for at least 5 years results in a greater persistence of effect than 2 to 3 years of therapy.[7–12] Discontinuation of risedronate following 3 years of treatment results in a more rapid loss of bone density and BTM than 2 years of alendronate or 3 years of zolendronate.[13,14]

Alendronate

When individuals were followed off of drug therapy following treatment with alendronate for 2 years or less, there were fewer robust effects on suppression of bone turnover and maintenance of BMD when compared with those for whom treatment with alendronate had been continued for 3 years or longer before discontinuation.[9–12]

Two cohorts of patients treated with alendronate for up to 10 years have been reported.[7,8] Both include an arm that saw placebo for 5 years following as many as 5 years of alendronate. In the Alendronate Phase III Osteoporosis Treatment Study Group, postmenopausal women with osteoporosis were randomized to alendronate 20 mg/d for 2 years followed by 5 mg/d for 1 year, 5 mg daily for 3 years, 10 mg daily for 3 years, or placebo.[15] Two 2-year extensions and then a 3-year extension were performed. The 5-mg and 10-mg daily arms continued on the same respective daily alendronate dose, whereas the placebo arm was discontinued after the first 2-year extension. The 20 mg/d × 2-years, 5 mg/d × 1-year original arm received 5 mg/d in the first 2-year extension (alendronate × 5 years) and then saw placebo for 5 years. Tonino and colleagues[16] reported the results of the second 2-year extension at year 7. For the alendronate × 5-years placebo × 2-years arm, no significant decline in BMD at the lumbar spine or hip was seen, but significant declines in the forearm were noted. Urinary N-telopeptide increased during the first year off therapy but then remained stable well below baseline (year 5 level −73%, year 7 level −57.9%). The 10-year results of this study were reported by Bone and colleagues,[7] in which this same group had now been followed off therapy for 5 years. BMD was maintained in the spine. Declines in BMD were noted in the total hip after year 7 (off therapy for 2 years) but at year 10 were comparable to those on alendronate 5 mg daily for the entire 10 years. Urine N-telopeptide remained suppressed at more than 50% of baseline levels.

The second alendronate cohort comes from FLEX, the Fracture Intervention Trial (FIT) Long Term Extension. In FIT, all patients received alendronate 5 mg/d for 2 years followed by 10 mg/d. Average follow-up was 2.9 years in the vertebral fracture arm and 4.2 years in the clinical fracture arm. Patients were offered up to 1 year of alendronate 10 mg/d on completion of FIT. FLEX enrolled 1099 patients who were then rerandomized to placebo (n = 437), alendronate 5 mg/d (n = 329), or alendronate 10 mg/d (n = 333), and followed for an 5 additional years. Patients in the placebo arm saw a 1.52% increase in lumbar spine BMD, with declines of 1.48% in the femoral neck, 3.38% in the total hip, and 3.21% in the forearm. The decline in BMD of the total hip exceeded the baseline value at the start of FLEX by 0.16%. BTM gradually increased over 5 years compared with those who remained on alendronate. When compared with pretreatment levels in FIT 10 years earlier, serum C-terminal telopeptide of type 1 collagen was −7% and N-propeptide of type 1 collagen was −24% in those who had been randomized to the placebo arm.[8]

Risedronate

In the VERT-NA (Vertebral Efficacy with Risedronate Therapy—North America) trial,[17] 599 of the 818 who completed the study were enrolled in a 1-year extension in which risedronate and placebo patients stopped therapy. Lumbar spine BMD decreased 0.83% and femoral neck BMD dropped 1.23% in those who had stopped risedronate, although these values were still greater than the control group who had been on placebo in the VERT-NA trial. Urine N-telopeptide increased significantly from a median of 30.3 nmol bone collagen equivalents (BCE)/mmol creatinine at end of treatment to 50.9 nmol BCE/mmol creatinine after 1 year off risedronate. This increase in the BTM represented a complete resolution of effect when compared with the control group.[13]

Ibandronate

There are no published data on the cessation of ibandronate and subsequent effects on BMD and BTM.

Zolendronate

Zolendronate, 5 mg is approved for every 24-month dosing in patients with osteopenia. In a study of 50 postmenopausal women with osteopenia, the effect of a single intravenous dose of 5 mg zolendronate persisted for the duration of a 3-year trial when compared with placebo control.[6] BMD was higher in the zolendronate group by 6.8% at the lumbar spine and 4.0% at the total hip. Mean levels of serum C-telopeptide were 44% lower than the placebo group.

The HORIZON PFT (Health Outcomes and Reduced Incidence with Zolendronic Acid Once Yearly Pivotal Fracture Trial) was a 3-year double-blind, placebo-controlled trial that enrolled 7736 postmenopausal women.[18] A 3-year extension of HORIZON PFT randomized 1233 women who had received intravenous zolendronate 5 mg yearly in the core trial to receive either 3 additional years of zolendronate[19] (Z6) or 3 years of placebo (Z3P3). The Z3P3 group saw declines of 2.03% in the lumbar spine, 1.2% in the total hip, and 1.04% in the femoral neck, values that were significant when compared with the Z6 group but still well above pretreatment levels. Markers of bone turnover "rose slightly" in the Z3P3 group but procollagen type 1 N-terminal pro-peptide remained "about 47% below" pretreatment values.[20]

Hormones

Estrogens have a waning effect on bone in postmenopausal women whether after short-term or long-term use. Short-term hormone therapy has been reported not to protect against bone loss after 1 or 2 years of discontinuation.[21–23] Long-term hormone therapy also failed to protect against bone loss. Evidence from the Framing-ham Study indicated that even after 7 years of estrogen therapy, there was little residual effect on bone density 10 to 20 years after estrogen withdrawal.[24,25]

The rate of bone loss from studies after estrogen withdrawal is still controversial. Some studies have reported identical bone loss rates compared with placebo, whereas others have reported accelerated bone loss versus placebo.[23] Some of the controversy is due to differences in study population (healthy or osteoporotic), duration of treatment and discontinuation periods, method of measuring bone mass changes, different treatment regimens, age of study population, and menopausal status.[23,26]

Raloxifene

The benefit of raloxifene for bone appears to be short lived after cessation of treatment. Naylor and colleagues[27] showed that the bone turnover response was lost 6 months after treatment cessation despite nearly 2 years of therapy. In addition, bone loss that was greater than in the control group, suggesting accelerated bone loss. Hip BMD was 2% less than baseline 192 weeks after treatment. Neele and colleagues[23] showed that 5 years of treatment with raloxifene did not protect against bone loss 1 year after withdrawal of therapy, and that the rate of bone loss was not significantly different from that of placebo-treated women.

Denosumab

Denosumab treatment has reversible characteristics that have been demonstrated in several clinical trials. In a study of osteopenic postmenopausal women, after treatment with denosumab (60 mg every 6 months × 4), cessation of therapy resulted in a return to baseline in serum C-telopeptide within 9 months followed by a compensatory overshoot at 12 months and return to baseline by 30 months after stopping denosumab.[28] BMD returned to baseline within 18 months of stopping the drug but remained above the BMD of the placebo treatment cohort.[12,28]

Teriparatide

BMD data were collected over an 18-month period after the conclusion of the Teriparatide Fracture Prevention trial. The BMD at the total hip and lumbar spine was maintained during this time, although it was somewhat confounded by the use of some osteoporosis medications such as bisphosphonates in 47% of those followed. The use of bisphosphonates for 12 months or more was associated with a greater maintenance of BMD gains than for those who did not use osteoporosis drugs.[29,30]

Similar results were seen in the lumbar spine BMD of men 30 months after stopping teriparatide.[31]

DISCONTINUATION OF OSTEOPOROSIS TREATMENT AND SUBSEQUENT FRACTURE RISK
Bisphosphonates

Studies suggest that a minimum of 2 to 3 years of bisphosphonate therapy with good compliance is needed to demonstrate fracture benefit. Furthermore, treatment with bisphosphonates for 3 to 5 years and subsequent discontinuation for 3 to 5 years is not associated with an increased risk of hip fracture (alendronate; zolendronate), but when compared to those who continued on bisphosphonate, is associated with increased risk of vertebral fractures (alendronate; zolendronate), and an increased risk of nonvertebral fractures in women without prevalent vertebral fractures and BMD T-scores of −2.5 or less (alendronate).

Information regarding the effects of discontinuation of bisphosphonates on fracture risk is limited, and drawing conclusions based on this is problematic. There are two sources of information that can be accessed: administrative databases and clinical trial extensions.

Gallagher and colleagues[32] studied 36,164 women in the General Practice Research Database (GPRD) in the United Kingdom who received a new prescription for alendronate (74.1%) or risedronate (25.9%). There was no evidence of residual effect on fracture risk after stopping bisphosphonate when the mean follow-up was 2.39 years, and few used bisphosphonates for 5 years of longer. Patients who recently stopped bisphosphonates had a similar fracture risk to those who had discontinued further in the past and to patients who had just started therapy.

New users of alendronate (77%) and risedronate (23%) were also the subject of a study by Curtis and colleagues.[33] In addition, they evaluated for the effect of compliance as measured by the medication possession ratio (MPR). A cohort of 9063 women who were members of "a large US healthcare organization" and compliant with drug therapy for at least 2 years were examined. Women who discontinued drug therapy had lower hip fracture rates than nonadherent women, if they had previously taken bisphosphonates for 2 or more years and had been compliant with drug therapy (MPR of 66%–100%). However, when time since discontinuation was examined, there was a twofold to threefold increased hazard ratio for hip fracture in women who had stopped more than 9 months ago. Women who discontinued drug therapy and who had higher degrees of compliance (MPR 88%–100%) and those previously having received bisphosphonates for 3 or more years had numerically lower rates of hip fracture than those who were less compliant or on shorter duration of drug therapy. Nevertheless, the fracture rates were still higher than those who remained on bisphosphonates.

A population-based, nested case-control study of women 68 years or older from Ontario, Canada recently looked at the incidence of subtrochanteric fracture in those on an oral bisphosphonate between 2002 and 2008. During this 6-year interval, short-term use of bisphosphonate (100 days to 3 years) did not reduce fracture risk, but use for 3 or more years did reduce fracture risk.[34]

Alendronate Clinical Extension Studies

The Alendronate Phase III Osteoporosis Treatment Study Group obtained lateral radiographs of the spine at the end of each extension. Morphometric vertebral fractures and clinical fractures were reported as safety end points. At 10 years, there was no evidence of an increased rate of morphometric vertebral fractures in the ALN5P5 discontinuation group (6.6%) as compared with the ALN10 (10 mg/d × 10 years) group (5.0%). During years 8 to 10, 12.0% of the ALN5P5 group sustained a first nonvertebral fracture compared with 8.1% in the ALN10 (10 mg) group and 11.5% in the ALN10 (5 mg) group.[7]

In the FLEX cohort, 437 patients who took alendronate 5 mg/d for 2 years then 10 mg/d for up to 3 years were randomized to placebo for 5 years. When compared with patients on 10 years of alendronate, clinical vertebral fractures were more common in the placebo group despite a slight increase in bone density in the spine over 5 years: placebo, 23 of 437 (5.3%) versus alendronate, 16 of 662 (2.4%) (95% confidence interval [CI] 0.24–0.85). A nonsignificant increase in morphometric fractures was also noted, but there was no difference in hip or nonvertebral fractures.[8]

A post hoc analysis of FLEX reported by Schwartz and colleagues[35] looked at those women without prevalent vertebral fractures at FLEX baseline, and found a greater risk of nonvertebral fractures in those who stopped alendronate after 5 years if their femoral neck T-score was −2.5 or less at FLEX baseline.

Risedronate Clinical Extension Studies

In the extension of VERT-NA, despite seeing significant declines in BMD and increases in BTM in the 1 year off risedronate, the incidence of new morphometric vertebral fractures was decreased by 46% compared with the placebo group (relative risk 0.54, 95% CI 0.34–0.86, $P = .009$). New vertebral fractures occurred in 26 of 398 (6.5%) patients who had previously taken risedronate and in 42 of 361 (11.6%) patients on placebo. By contrast, there was no significant difference in nonvertebral fractures, with 19 of 398 (4.8%) in the risedronate group and 18 of 361 (5.0%) in the placebo group (although these were collected as adverse events and radiologic confirmation was not required).[13] This result suggests a residual protective effect of risedronate on morphometric fractures but, because there was not a comparator group that continued on risedronate, questions as to diminished fracture benefit associated with drug holiday cannot be addressed.

Zolendronate Clinical Extension Studies

In the 3-year extension of the HORIZON PFT trial, with more modest declines in BMD and slight increases in BTM, new morphometric vertebral fractures occurred more frequently in the Z3P3 group compared with those who continued on zolendronate (Z6). There were 30 fractures in 486 patients (6.2%) in the Z3P3 group and 14 fractures in 469 patients (3.0%) in the Z6 group (hazard ratio 2.07, $P = .04$). However, there were no reported differences in the rate of clinical vertebral, hip, and nonvertebral fractures between the Z3P3 and Z6 groups.[20]

Hormone Therapy

Case-control studies have suggested a minimum of 5 years of estrogen treatment to reduce fracture risk.[26] The Women's Health Initiative (WHI) noted a 33% reduction in hip fractures in healthy postmenopausal women (not just women with osteoporosis) who had been treated with estrogen therapy for an average of 5.6 years.[36] However, estrogens have been relegated to short-term use at the lowest possible dose to alleviate menopause symptoms, not for the prevention of chronic disease.[37,38] Studies of fracture risk after cessation of estrogen have noted a loss in fracture risk protection.[36,38–40] The FDA no longer recommends estrogen therapy for the treatment of osteoporosis.

Raloxifene

Raloxifene has been shown to be effective in preventing postmenopausal bone loss and vertebral fractures over a 3-year period in the randomized double-blind MORE trial (Multiple Outcomes of Raloxifene Evaluation) and the 3-year continuation with the CORE trial (Continuing Outcomes Relevant to Evista). This trial ultimately produced 8 years of safety data with raloxifene use and no significant change in fracture data, including no significant reduction in hip fracture risk compared with placebo.[27,41,42] There is no limit on duration of treatment with raloxifene. Significant declines in bone density occur shortly after cessation of raloxifene therapy.[43] However, there are no data on the change in fracture risk after discontinuing raloxifene.

Denosumab

Denosumab, given subcutaneously twice yearly for 3 years, was associated with a reduction in the risk of vertebral, nonvertebral, and hip fractures in women with osteoporosis.[44] Six years of continuous treatment was associated with continued BMD accrual.[45] The original pivotal fracture trial will be expanded through a 7-year extension, which will provide 10 years of data regarding long-term efficacy and safety. There is currently no recommended limit on duration of denosumab therapy.

There have not been sufficiently large studies to clarify fracture rates after stopping denosumab treatment in comparison with placebo. However, in the BTM and BMD study previously noted, there were no fracture rate differences in the 2-year period after 2 years of treatment compared with placebo: 3% nonvertebral fractures in each group and no clinical vertebral fractures were reported.[28]

Teriparatide

In the Fracture Prevention Trial (FPT), treatment with once-daily teriparatide significantly reduced the risk of vertebral and nonvertebral fractures over a median duration of observation of 21 months.[46] Lindsay and colleagues[19] concluded that increased duration of teriparatide therapy resulted in a progressive decrease in the rate of nonvertebral fragility fractures and back pain, and adverse events occurred early in the treatment and not later, thus suggesting that patients may achieve improved outcomes by persisting on teriparatide therapy.

Expert review of the finding of osteosarcoma in teriparatide-treated Fischer 344 rats indicated that this finding was unlikely to predict an increased risk of osteosarcoma in human patients receiving teriparatide treatment for up to 2 years. Therefore in the United States, approval by the FDA was for 2 years of treatment.[30] Further efficacy and safety was found in glucocorticoid-treated subjects considered at high risk of fracture when treated with 3 years of teriparatide therapy; nevertheless, the FDA has not altered the recommended treatment interval of 2 years.[47]

There were 18 months of follow-up after the cessation of teriparatide in the FPT. Although there was confounding with bisphosphonate use, there was a continued significant fracture reduction effect that continued during this period, independent of bisphosphonate use, according to a logistic regression analysis.[29,30] Again this was similar to the continued vertebral fracture efficacy in males up to 30 months after cessation of teriparatide treatment.[31]

DECIDING WHAT TO DO WITH PATIENTS; WHAT TO MAKE OF REPORTS OF ATYPICAL FRACTURES IN PATIENTS ON LONG-TERM BISPHOSPHONATES?

Among the drugs approved for treatment of postmenopausal osteoporosis, only the bisphosphonates have demonstrated suppression of BTM and maintenance of

BMD for more than 12 to 18 months after a drug is withdrawn. This finding is consistent with their unique mechanism of action in binding to hydroxyapatite in bone. Moreover, the presence of atypical fractures has to date only been linked to patients treated with bisphosphonates. Therefore, at present the concept of drug holiday, whereby one might maintain fracture risk reduction while minimizing adverse events, is really only applicable to bisphosphonates.

Among the bisphosphonates, there are no current studies that demonstrate comparable across-the-board fracture benefit for those who discontinue the drug as opposed to those who continue on treatment, for whom length of therapy is at least 3 to 5 years before cessation. Therefore, for those at sufficiently high risk for fracture, a decision as to whether to continue drug therapy is based on the perception of risk of drug side effects.

Of the side effects reported to be associated with long-term bisphosphonate use, namely ONJ and atypical subtrochanteric femoral shaft fractures (SFSF), ONJ appears to occur less frequently in the postmenopausal population, with a prevalence of 1 in 10,000 to 1 in 100,000.

Schilcher and Aspenberg[48] noted an SFSF incident density of 1 per 1000 patient-years in a defined health care registry in Sweden, with a mean duration of exposure of 5.8 years (range 3.5–8.5 years). Dell and colleagues[49,50] noted an SFSF incidence of 0.02 per 1000 patient-years for the first 2 years and 0.78 per 1000 patient-years for 8 years of bisphosphonate therapy in a study of patients seen in the Kaiser Permanente health care system in California. In both of these studies, radiographs were individually reviewed for features of atypia. By contrast, Park-Wyllie relied on ICD-9 codes for the diagnosis of subtrochanteric and femoral shaft fractures, and identified an increased risk of 1.35 per 1000 patients in those on bisphosphonates for 6 years and 2.22 per 1000 patients for those on treatment for 7 years.[34] Using the population of women studied in FIT, the risk for osteoporotic fracture is 10-to 23-fold greater than for SFSF for women with a prior vertebral fracture, and 7- to 10-fold greater in those without a prevalent vertebral fracture.[49,51]

Two recent studies have looked at larger populations to attempt to overcome issues related to the small number of cases of SFSF. Schilcher and colleagues[52] reviewed all 1234 radiographs of femoral subtrochanteric or shaft fractures reported in the 2008 National Swedish Patient Register, and linked this to patient history and medication use. The age-adjusted relative risk of atypical fracture with any use of bisphosphonate was 47.3 (95% CI 25.6–87.3) with a number needed to harm of 1 case per 2000 patients per year of bisphosphonate use. Wang and Bhattacharyya[53] used the Nationwide Inpatient Sample (NIS) to examine 90 million hospital discharge records in men and women older than 65 years between 1996 and 2007, and the Medical Expenditure Panel Survey to estimate rates of medication use. In the setting of an increase in bisphosphonate use in women from 3.5% to 16.6%, there was a decline in hospitalization for typical osteoporotic hip fractures of greater than 30,000, with a small but significant increase of 2500 subtrochanteric fractures. Using age-adjusted rates, the investigators estimated that for every 100 typical osteoporotic hip fractures prevented by bisphosphonate use, there was an increase of 1 atypical subtrochanteric fracture.

Thus all recent studies demonstrate that the risk-benefit ratio favors drug therapy in those postmenopausal women at risk for osteoporotic fracture. However, effectively communicating this to patients is hampered by several factors. Numeracy—the ability to understand numbers—is remarkably limited.[54] In one study 16% of highly educated people incorrectly answered simple questions about risk magnitude, such as which represents the larger risk: 1%, 5%, or 10%? Presenting absolute risk (eg, among users of bisphosphonates, 1 patient out of 1000 will have an atypical fracture) increases comprehension over relative risk (eg, 46% greater likelihood of an atypical fracture in bisphosphonate users vs nonusers).[54] Numerous other factors also influence risk perception. Newly discovered risk (eg, recent news reports of spontaneous femoral fractures) may be perceived as a greater risk than those that are well established. A dreaded risk (eg, spontaneously fracturing your femur while walking down the hall) is also overestimated.[54,55]

An Alternative Form of Drug Holiday: Switching from Bisphosphonate to Teriparatide

Theoretically, the switch from a bisphosphonate to an anabolic drug such as teriparatide might undo the suppressive effects of bisphosphonates on bone and lower the risk of SFSF. In a small study of 38 postmenopausal women who had been on bisphosphonates for a mean duration of approximately 5 years, 24 months of teriparatide (20 µg/d) reduced microdamage accumulation seen on iliac crest biopsies compared with a placebo group that had not previously seen a bisphosphonate.[56] In postmenopausal women with osteoporosis based on BMD, 2 years of teriparatide increased bone formation (based on biopsy and biochemical markers) to a comparable level in both treatment-naïve patients and individuals previously treated with alendronate for a mean of slightly longer than 5 years.[57] In addition, 1 year of teriparatide following at least 2 years of alendronate or risedronate therapy demonstrated an increase in heterogeneity in BMD distribution, as measured on paired iliac crest bone biopsies obtained before and after teriparatide therapy.[58]

An Algorithm for Patients Already on Drug Therapy

Given the limitations with available data, an approach when discussing "how long to treat" with individual patients is to first categorize their fracture risk (low, intermediate, high). This gradation can be based on a clinical assessment that includes but is not limited to fracture history, age, BMD (spine and hip; changes over time), FRAX, and frailty including frequency of falls. There are no universally accepted criteria to stratify according to risk, and a variety of approaches exist.[4,5,59,60]

Five years can be a decision point, because most case reports of SFSF were on bisphosphonates for at least that long, and the limited number of extension studies saw bisphosphonates for 3 to 5 years before going on to placebo.

Then, gauge the patient's "risk profile": are they more concerned about risk of drug side effects or the risk of fracture? This usually becomes apparent in a discussion about ONJ and SFSF in the setting of bisphosphonate use.

This algorithm would not be applicable to patients with poor compliance on oral bisphosphonates, or those who have had clear evidence of a significant decline in bone density while on bisphosphonate therapy. It is assumed that these patients are not seeing the suppressive effects on bone turnover that may lead to SFSF.

For Patients at Very Low Risk for Fracture

This category is based on FRAX and clinical assessment (no evidence of accelerated bone loss; without frequent falls). This category would include many patients originally started on drug therapy for "prevention," for example.

- Bisphosphonates can be stopped until fracture risk is increased
- Evista can be continued for at least 5 to 10 years[61] to prevent bone loss and lower risk of invasive breast cancer
- Hormone therapy: use lowest possible dose for shortest possible time.

For Patients at Intermediate Risk for Fracture

Individuals no prior fragility fractures as an adult, are osteopenic on BMD, but whose FRAX 10-year risk for fracture meets National Osteoporosis Foundation (NOF) guidelines for treatment.

- Bisphosphonates
  - Assess patient's risk tolerance:
    - Concerned about drug side effects > risk for fragility fracture
      - Bisphosphonates can be used for 5 years with periodic check of oral health and thigh pain
        - Then stop for drug holiday of several years
        - Monitor bone density every 2 years and BTM yearly
        - Resume therapy if significant declines in BMD, significant increase in BTM, or new interval fractures
    - Concerned about risk for fracture > drug side effects
      - Continue on drug therapy monitoring oral health and thigh pain
- Raloxifene: can be continued for at least 5 to 10 years[61] to prevent bone loss and lower risk of invasive breast cancer
- Hormone therapy: not recommended long term.

For Patients at High Risk for Fracture

Individuals with prior fragility fractures, FRAX 10-year risk for fracture that exceeds NOF guidelines for treatment; or very low BMD (−3.0 or <) without prior fracture.

- Bisphosphonates can be used for at least 10 years with periodic check for oral health and thigh pain
  - If no prior teriparatide therapy or contraindications, consider switching to 2 years of teriparatide for drug holiday from bisphosphonates
  - If opposed then:
    - Assess patient's risk averseness
      - Concerned about drug side effects > risk for fracture
        - Stop for drug holiday of several years
        - Monitor bone density every 2 years and BTM yearly
        - Resume therapy if significant declines in BMD or greater than 40% increase in BTM
      - Concerned about risk for fracture > drug side effects
        - Continue on drug therapy monitoring oral health and thigh pain
- Denosumab: monitor for ONJ and SFSF
- Teriparatide for 2 years followed by yearly intravenous bisphosphonate or denosumab.

Patients with Documented Atypical Subtrochanteric Fracture on Bisphosphonate

- Stop bisphosphonate
- Evaluate for stress reaction on contralateral femur
- Consider teriparatide for 2 years; subsequent intravenous zolendronate perhaps less often than yearly, or denosumab.

SUMMARY

In providing recommendations to patients regarding drug therapy, the health care provider must balance drug efficacy with side effects against drug therapy. Thus the FDA defines "safe" as meaning that the benefit outweighs the risk. For the postmenopausal woman with low bone mass, the question is one of relative risk: is the risk of fragility fracture greater than the risk of drug side effect?

There are no current studies that demonstrate comparable across-the-board fracture benefit for those who discontinue a drug as opposed to those who continue on treatment, for whom length of therapy is 3 to 5 years before cessation. The residual effect on BMD and BTM during the "holiday" after cessation of bisphosphonate treatment implies ongoing fracture risk reduction, but such a benefit has not been definitively established. Therefore, for those at sufficiently high risk for fracture, a decision as to whether to continue on drug therapy is based on the perception of the risk of drug side effects.

REFERENCES

1. Russell RG, Watts NB, Ebetino FH, et al. Mechanisms of action of bisphosphonates: similarities and differences and their potential influence on clinical efficacy. Osteoporos Int 2008;19(6):733–59.
2. Kennel KA, Drake MT. Adverse effects of bisphosphonates: implications for osteoporosis management. Mayo Clin Proc 2009;84(7):632–7 [quiz: 638].
3. Nancollas GH, Tang R, Phipps RJ, et al. Novel insights into actions of bisphosphonates on bone: differences in interactions with hydroxyapatite. Bone 2006;38(5): 617–27.
4. Seeman E. To stop or not to stop, that is the question. Osteoporos Int 2009;20(2): 187–95.
5. Watts NB, Diab DL. Long-term use of bisphosphonates in osteoporosis. J Clin Endocrinol Metab 2010;95(4):1555–65.
6. Grey A, Bolland M, Wattie D, et al. Prolonged antiresorptive activity of zoledronate: a randomized, controlled trial. J Bone Miner Res 2010;25(10):2251–5.
7. Bone HG, Hosking D, Devogelaer JP, et al. Ten years' experience with alendronate for osteoporosis in postmenopausal women. N Engl J Med 2004;350(12): 1189–99.
8. Black DM, Schwartz AV, Ensrud KE, et al. Effects of continuing or stopping alendronate after 5 years of treatment: the Fracture Intervention Trial Long-term Extension (FLEX): a randomized trial. JAMA 2006;296(24):2927–38.
9. Stock JL, Bell NH, Chesnut CH 3rd, et al. Increments in bone mineral density of the lumbar spine and hip and suppression of bone turnover are maintained after discontinuation of alendronate in postmenopausal women. Am J Med 1997; 103(4):291–7.
10. Rossini M, Gatti D, Zamberlan N, et al. Long-term effects of a treatment course with oral alendronate of postmenopausal osteoporosis. J Bone Miner Res 1994; 9(11):1833–7.
11. Greenspan SL, Emkey RD, Bone HG, et al. Significant differential effects of alendronate, estrogen, or combination therapy on the rate of bone loss after discontinuation of treatment of postmenopausal osteoporosis. A randomized, double-blind, placebo-controlled trial. Ann Intern Med 2002;137(11):875–83.
12. Miller PD, Bolognese MA, Lewiecki EM, et al. Effect of denosumab on bone density and turnover in postmenopausal women with low bone mass after long-term continued, discontinued, and restarting of therapy: a randomized blinded phase 2 clinical trial. Bone 2008;43(2):222–9.
13. Watts NB, Chines A, Olszynski WP, et al. Fracture risk remains reduced one year after discontinuation of risedronate. Osteoporos Int 2008;19(3):365–72.

14. Black D, Reid I, Cauley J, et al. The effect of 3 versus 6 years of zoledronic acid treatment in osteoporosis: a randomized extension to the HORIZON-pivotal fracture trial. J Bone Miner Res 2010;25(Suppl 1):S22 [abstract:1070].
15. Liberman UA, Weiss SR, Broll J, et al. Effect of oral alendronate on bone mineral density and the incidence of fractures in postmenopausal osteoporosis. The Alendronate Phase III Osteoporosis Treatment Study Group. N Engl J Med 1995;333(22):1437–43.
16. Tonino RP, Meunier PJ, Emkey R, et al. Skeletal benefits of alendronate: 7-year treatment of postmenopausal osteoporotic women. Phase III Osteoporosis Treatment Study Group. J Clin Endocrinol Metab 2000;85(9):3109–15.
17. Harris ST, Watts NB, Genant HK, et al. Effects of risedronate treatment on vertebral and nonvertebral fractures in women with postmenopausal osteoporosis: a randomized controlled trial. Vertebral Efficacy With Risedronate Therapy (VERT) Study Group. JAMA 1999;282(14):1344–52.
18. Black DM, Delmas PD, Eastell R, et al. Once-yearly zoledronic acid for treatment of postmenopausal osteoporosis. N Engl J Med 2007;356(18):1809–22.
19. Lindsay R, Miller P, Pohl G, et al. Relationship between duration of teriparatide therapy and clinical outcomes in postmenopausal women with osteoporosis. Osteoporos Int 2009;20(6):943–8.
20. Black D, Reid I, Cauley J, et al. The effect of 3 versus 6 years of zolendronic acid treatment in osteoporosis: a randomized extension in the HORIZON-pivotal fracture trial (PFT). J Bone Miner Res 2010.
21. Christiansen C, Christensen MS, Transbol I. Bone mass after withdrawal of oestrogen replacement. Lancet 1981;1(8228):1053–4.
22. Christiansen C, Christensen MS, Transbol I. Bone mass in postmenopausal women after withdrawal of oestrogen/gestagen replacement therapy. Lancet 1981;1(8218):459–61.
23. Neele SJ, Evertz R, De Valk-De Roo G, et al. Effect of 1 year of discontinuation of raloxifene or estrogen therapy on bone mineral density after 5 years of treatment in healthy postmenopausal women. Bone 2002;30(4):599–603.
24. Ettinger B, Grady D. The waning effect of postmenopausal estrogen therapy on osteoporosis. N Engl J Med 1993;329(16):1192–3.
25. Felson DT, Zhang Y, Hannan MT, et al. The effect of postmenopausal estrogen therapy on bone density in elderly women. N Engl J Med 1993;329(16):1141–6.
26. Tremollieres FA, Pouilles JM, Ribot C. Withdrawal of hormone replacement therapy is associated with significant vertebral bone loss in postmenopausal women. Osteoporos Int 2001;12(5):385–90.
27. Naylor KE, Clowes JA, Finigan J, et al. The effect of cessation of raloxifene treatment on bone turnover in postmenopausal women. Bone 2010;46(3):592–7.
28. Bone HG, Bolognese MA, Yuen CK, et al. Effects of denosumab treatment and discontinuation on bone mineral density and bone turnover markers in postmenopausal women with low bone mass. J Clin Endocrinol Metab 2011;96(4):972–80.
29. Prince R, Sipos A, Hossain A, et al. Sustained nonvertebral fragility fracture risk reduction after discontinuation of teriparatide treatment. J Bone Miner Res 2005;20(9):1507–13.
30. Lindsay R, Scheele WH, Neer R, et al. Sustained vertebral fracture risk reduction after withdrawal of teriparatide in postmenopausal women with osteoporosis. Arch Intern Med 2004;164(18):2024–30.
31. Kaufman JM, Orwoll E, Goemaere S, et al. Teriparatide effects on vertebral fractures and bone mineral density in men with osteoporosis: treatment and discontinuation of therapy. Osteoporos Int 2005;16(5):510–6.

32. Gallagher AM, Rietbrock S, Olson M, et al. Fracture outcomes related to persistence and compliance with oral bisphosphonates. J Bone Miner Res 2008;23(10): 1569–75.

33. Curtis JR, Westfall AO, Cheng H, et al. Risk of hip fracture after bisphosphonate discontinuation: implications for a drug holiday. Osteoporos Int 2008;19(11): 1613–20.

34. Park-Wyllie LY, Mamdani MM, Juurlink DN, et al. Bisphosphonate use and the risk of subtrochanteric or femoral shaft fractures in older women. JAMA 2011;305(8): 783–9.

35. Schwartz AV, Bauer DC, Cummings SR, et al. Efficacy of continued alendronate for fractures in women with and without prevalent vertebral fracture: the FLEX trial. J Bone Miner Res 2010;25(5):976–82.

36. Shifren JL, Schiff I. Role of hormone therapy in the management of menopause. Obstet Gynecol 2010;115(4):839–55.

37. Rossouw JE, Anderson GL, Prentice RL, et al. Risks and benefits of estrogen plus progestin in healthy postmenopausal women: principal results from the Women's Health Initiative randomized controlled trial. JAMA 2002;288(3):321–33.

38. Wasnich RD, Bagger YZ, Hosking DJ, et al. Changes in bone density and turnover after alendronate or estrogen withdrawal. Menopause 2004;11(6 Pt 1): 622–30.

39. Ascott-Evans BH, Guanabens N, Kivinen S, et al. Alendronate prevents loss of bone density associated with discontinuation of hormone replacement therapy: a randomized controlled trial. Arch Intern Med 2003;163(7):789–94.

40. Yates J, Barrett-Connor E, Barlas S, et al. Rapid loss of hip fracture protection after estrogen cessation: evidence from the National Osteoporosis Risk Assessment. Obstet Gynecol 2004;103(3):440–6.

41. Martino S, Disch D, Dowsett SA, et al. Safety assessment of raloxifene over eight years in a clinical trial setting. Curr Med Res Opin 2005;21(9):1441–52.

42. Olevsky OM, Martino S. Randomized clinical trials of raloxifene: reducing the risk of osteoporosis and breast cancer in postmenopausal women. Menopause 2008; 15(Suppl 4):790–6.

43. Briot K, Tremollieres F, Thomas T, et al. How long should patients take medications for postmenopausal osteoporosis? Joint Bone Spine 2007;74(1):24–31.

44. Cummings SR, San Martin J, McClung MR, et al. Denosumab for prevention of fractures in postmenopausal women with osteoporosis. N Engl J Med 2009; 361(8):756–65.

45. Miller PD, Wagman RB, Peacock M, et al. Effect of denosumab on bone mineral density and biochemical markers of bone turnover: six-year results of a phase 2 clinical trial. J Clin Endocrinol Metab 2011;96(2):394–402.

46. Neer RM, Arnaud CD, Zanchetta JR, et al. Effect of parathyroid hormone (1-34) on fractures and bone mineral density in postmenopausal women with osteoporosis. N Engl J Med 2001;344(19):1434–41.

47. Saag KG, Zanchetta JR, Devogelaer JP, et al. Effects of teriparatide versus alendronate for treating glucocorticoid-induced osteoporosis: thirty-six-month results of a randomized, double-blind, controlled trial. Arthritis Rheum 2009; 60(11):3346–55.

48. Schilcher J, Aspenberg P. Incidence of stress fractures of the femoral shaft in women treated with bisphosphonate. Acta Orthop 2009;80(4):413–5.

49. Dell R, Greene D, Ott S, et al. A retrospective analysis of all atypical femur fractures seen in a large California HMO from the years 2007 to 2009. ASBMR Annual Meeting. Toronto, Canada, 2010. p. S61 [abstract: 1201].

50. Shane E, Burr D, Ebeling PR, et al. Atypical subtrochanteric and diaphyseal femoral fractures: report of a task force of the American Society for Bone and Mineral Research. J Bone Miner Res 2010;25(11):2267–94.
51. Black DM, Kelly MP, Genant HK, et al. Bisphosphonates and fractures of the subtrochanteric or diaphyseal femur. N Engl J Med 2010;362(19):1761–71.
52. Schilcher J, Michaelsson K, Aspenberg P. Bisphosphonate use and atypical fractures of the femoral shaft. N Engl J Med 2011;364(18):1728–37.
53. Wang Z, Bhattacharyya T. Trends in incidence of subtrochanteric fragility fractures and bisphosphonate use among the US elderly, 1996–2007. J Bone Miner Res 2011;26(3):553–60.
54. Peters E, Hibbard J, Slovic P, et al. Numeracy skill and the communication, comprehension, and use of risk-benefit information. Health Aff (Millwood) 2007; 26(3):741–8.
55. Cohen JT, Neumann PJ. What's more dangerous, your aspirin or your car? Thinking rationally about drug risks (and benefits). Health Aff (Millwood) 2007; 26(3):636–46.
56. Dobnig H, Stepan JJ, Burr DB, et al. Teriparatide reduces bone microdamage accumulation in postmenopausal women previously treated with alendronate. J Bone Miner Res 2009;24(12):1998–2006.
57. Stepan JJ, Burr DB, Li J, et al. Histomorphometric changes by teriparatide in alendronate-pretreated women with osteoporosis. Osteoporos Int 2010;21(12): 2027–36.
58. Misof BM, Paschalis EP, Blouin S, et al. Effects of 1 year of daily teriparatide treatment on iliacal bone mineralization density distribution (BMDD) in postmenopausal osteoporotic women previously treated with alendronate or risedronate. J Bone Miner Res 2010;25(11):2297–303.
59. Leslie WD, Morin S, Lix LM. A before-and-after study of fracture risk reporting and osteoporosis treatment initiation. Ann Intern Med 2010;153(9):580–6.
60. Davis SR, Kirby C, Weekes A, et al. Simplifying screening for osteoporosis in Australian primary care: the Prospective Screening for Osteoporosis; Australian Primary Care Evaluation of Clinical Tests (PROSPECT) study. Menopause 2011; 18(1):53–9.
61. Sambrook P. Who will benefit from treatment with selective estrogen receptor modulators (SERMs)? Best Pract Res Clin Rheumatol 2005;19(6):975–81.

Emerging Therapies for Osteoporosis

Chad Deal, MD[a,b]

KEYWORDS

- Cathepsin K • Sclerostin • Osteoporosis • Serotonin
- Wnt signaling

The bone remodeling unit (BRU) comprises a well-choreographed sequence of events, during which osteoclasts resorb bone during a period of about 3 weeks, creating resorption cavities that are collectively termed the remodeling space. Resorption is followed by osteoblast activation and formation of osteoid, which fill the cavities in a period of about 3 months. Primary and secondary mineralization follow (**Fig. 1**). When active matrix synthesis is finished, osteoblasts become embedded in the matrix and function as osteocytes (**Fig. 2**). These cells remain active in bone remodeling by maintaining connections to the bone surface, the BRU, and to other osteocytes via an extensive canalicular network. Fluid flows through this network and is believed to be able to induce signaling that allows osteocytes to function as mechanoreceptors that direct remodeling to areas that require repair and are important regulators of mineralization.[1,2] Bone remodeling is an active and dynamic process and interventions that limit resorption (antiresorptive therapy) or augment formation (anabolic therapy) allow for effective treatment of bone loss and low bone mass (LBM).[3]

Treatment with antiresorptive agents eventually leads to a decrease in osteoblast function. The initial increase in bone mass resulting from the use of this type of therapy occurs because of inhibition of bone resorption by osteoclasts while osteoblasts continue to function and fill in the remodeling space. This uncoupling of formation and resorption is time limited (1–2 years) before osteoblast function declines and increases in bone mass begin to slow. Subsequent increases in bone mass are largely related to an increase in mineralization density, a result of reduced bone turnover and aging bone. The only known anabolic agent, teriparatide (TPTD), is limited to 24 months in the United States and 18 months in Europe because of the development of osteosarcoma in an animal toxicology study that resulted in discontinuation of the clinical trial after a mean treatment duration of 19 months.[4] Since its release in 2002, TPTD does not seem to be associated with the development of osteosarcoma

[a] Orthopedic and Rheumatology Institute, Department of Rheumatology, Center for Osteoporosis and Metabolic Bone Disease, Cleveland, OH, USA
[b] Clinic Lerner College of Medicine at Case Western Reserve University, Cleveland Clinic, 9500 Euclid Avenue, A50, Cleveland, OH 44195, USA
E-mail address: dealc@ccf.org

Rheum Dis Clin N Am 37 (2011) 337–350
doi:10.1016/j.rdc.2011.07.006
0889-857X/11/$ – see front matter © 2011 Elsevier Inc. All rights reserved.

rheumatic.theclinics.com

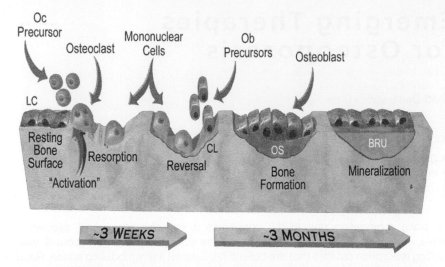

LC = Lining Cells   CL = Cement Line   OS = Osteoid   BRU = Bone Remodeling Unit

Fig. 1. The sequence of bone remodeling in healthy individuals. Remodeling is initiated when osteoclasts are activated, resorb bone, and create resorption cavities. Resorption is followed by osteoblast activation and formation of osteoid, which fills in the resorption cavity. Primary and secondary mineralization follow and continue for years. The active and dynamic process of bone remodeling is the target for pharmaceutical agents that affect bone resorption and formation. Ob, osteoblast; Oc, osteoclast.

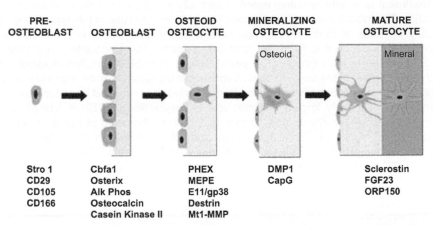

Fig. 2. Marker expression osteoblast to osteocyte ontogeny. Osteocytes are likely descendants of matrix-producing osteoblasts. Some osteoblasts embed in the matrix and extend projections that develop into the canicular system. This system is critical for osteocyte communication with bone cells and for mechanoreceptor function. The signals that are important for osteoblast and osteocyte development are shown as well as secretory products of osteocytes including the Wnt inhibitor sclerostin, which is an exclusive product of osteocytes. (*From* Bonewald L. The amazing osteocyte. J Bone Miner Res 2011;26:231; with permission.)

in humans. There have been case reports of osteosarcoma occurring in patients treated with teriparatide.[5] Based on the numbers of patients treated with TPTD and the background incidence of osteosarcoma in the population, more than 2 cases would be expected.

Research is currently focusing on drugs that target the remodeling cycle by affecting osteoblasts, osteoclasts, and osteocytes, and/or molecules that control signaling pathways important for cell function and gene transcription. The role of serotonin in control of bone mass is emerging. This article reviews the types and modes of action of therapies that are in development for the treatment of patients with LBM.

ANTIRESORPTIVE AGENTS

Bisphosphonates are the most frequently used antiresorptive agents. These drugs bind avidly to hydroxyapatite and work by inhibiting farnesyl pyrophosphate synthase, an enzyme in the mevalonate pathway.[6] This pathway is important for protein prenylation, the attachment of lipids to proteins, which is critical for cytoskeletal organization in osteoclasts. Inhibition of the pathway disrupts cytoskeletal structure, which prevents osteoclasts from being able to form a ruffled border on the bone during the remodeling process, generate a proton gradient, and resorb mineral and matrix.

Bone resorption and formation are tightly coupled. As described earlier, inhibition of resorption eventually results in inhibition of formation. An agent that inhibits bone resorption but allows bone formation to continue would, therefore, have a greater effect on bone mass and bone quality than currently available agents. This uncoupling of formation and resorption occurs in mice and humans with an osteopetrosis phenotype characterized by the absence of the chloride 7 channel, a membrane complex that is required to generate an acid milieu in the resorption lacunae. There is ongoing bone formation despite the absence of functional osteoclasts and reduced bone resorption.[7]

Cathepsin K Inhibitors

Osteoclasts are specialized cells that effect bone resorption. Bone resorption requires dissolution of the mineral components and removal of organic bone matrix. Demineralization requires acid secretion by osteoclasts into resorption lacunae, whereas matrix degradation is accomplished by cysteine proteases including cathepsins (**Fig. 3**).[8] Eleven cathepsins have been identified. Cathepsin K, a cysteine protease produced by osteoclasts, is the most important because it has potent collagenase activity in acidic environments such as the resorption lacunae.[9] Pycnodysostosis is a rare disease characterized by high bone mass (HBM) acroosteolysis of distal phalanxes, short stature, and cranial deformities. It results from a genetic mutation resulting in loss of function of the cathepsin K gene.[10] Elimination of cathepsin K in osteoclasts results in inhibition of bone resorption. Drugs that inhibit cathepsin K are suggested to have less effect on osteoclast-osteoblast interaction because they do not result in osteoclast apoptosis as do bisphosphonates. Human cathepsin K inhibitors have been shown to prevent bone loss in ovariectomized mice without blunting the anabolic action of parathyroid hormone (PTH).[11] Odanacatib inactivates the proteolytic activity of cathepsin K, is selective for cathepsin K, and does not result in accumulation of abnormal collagen in fibroblasts as seen with other cathepsin inhibitors. Cathepsin inhibitors other than odanacatib seem less specific for cathepsin K and have been associated with skin reactions. This finding has resulted in suspension of drug development of all cathepsin K except for odanacatib. Inhibition of cathepsin K in humans by this orally bioavailable agent is being evaluated in several ongoing trials.

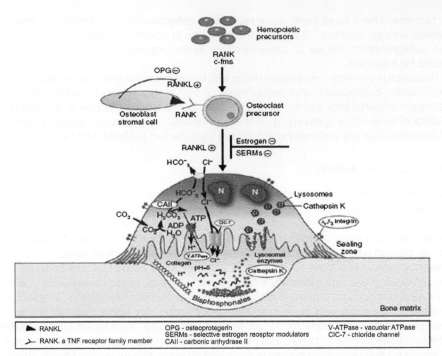

Fig. 3. Maturation of precursors to osteoclasts and the intracellular pathways in osteoclast function. Odanacatib inhibits the formation of cathepsin K and reduces matrix degradation.

The 24-month results of a randomized, controlled trial (RCT) of 399 postmenopausal women with T-scores between −2.0 and −3.5 at the lumbar spine or hip sites has been reported.[12] Four doses of odanacatib given as a weekly oral dose were evaluated and showed dose-dependent increases in bone density of the spine (+5.7%), total hip (+4.1%), femoral neck (+4.7%), and radius (+2.9%). Although urine *N*-telopeptide of type I collagen, a marker of bone resorption, declined 52%, bone-specific alkaline phosphatase, a marker of bone formation, declined only 13% (decline with placebo was −3%). This finding suggests less inhibition of bone formation than is found with current antiresorptive therapies. The drug was generally safe and well tolerated with no dose-related trends in adverse events including rashes. An extension study to 36 months enrolled 189 patients and compared the 50-mg weekly dose with placebo. Lumbar spine density increases from baseline and from year 2 to year 3 were 7.9% and 2.3%, whereas total hip increased 5.8% and 2.4% respectively **(Fig. 4)**.[13] For those continuing therapy, markers of bone formation remained near baseline. After discontinuation of odanacatib, bone density declined at all sites and at year 3 lumbar spine density was only +1.4% more than the baseline value at study initiation, total hip density was −0.5% less than baseline. This decline was more rapid than occurs after discontinuation of bisphosphonate therapy. Markers of bone resorption increased to more than 50% more than baseline after discontinuation of odanacatib but returned to baseline by month 36 **(Fig. 5)**. Markers of bone formation also increased. This drug, like the recently released denosumab, has what could be termed a rapid resolution of effect, whereas bisphosphonates have a more prolonged resolution of effect.[14] Rapid resolution of effect might be preferable in some clinical settings including the prevention of a blunting effect of the first therapy when subsequent

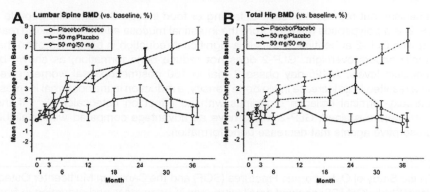

Fig. 4. Mean percent change from baseline more than 3 years for bone mineral density (BMD) at the lumbar spine (*A*) and total hip (*B*) with 3 years of odanacatib and 2 years of odanacatib and 1 year of placebo. (*From* Eisman J, Bone HG, Hosking DJ, et al. Odanacatib in the treatment of postmenopausal women with low bone mineral density: three-year continued therapy and resolution of effect. J Bone Miner Res 2011;26:246; with permission.)

treatment is initiated, if long term side effects are a concern, or in women of child-bearing potential. However, interruptions in therapy and poor compliance may have a more rapid loss of bone mass and fracture effect. The fracture trial results for oda-nacatib are expected in 2012 (clinicaltrails.gov NCT00529373).

Glucagonlike Peptide 2

Glucagonlike peptide is an intestinal hormone released in response to food intake. Bone remodeling has a circadian rhythm with a nocturnal increase in bone resorption.[15] This circadian rhythm is affected by food intake. The circadian variation seen in humans, high in the morning and low in the evening, may not be an inherent

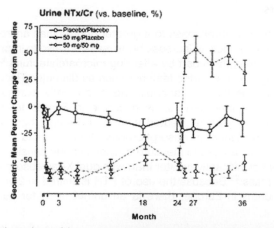

Fig. 5. Biochemical marker of bone resorption, urine NTx expressed as geometric mean change from baseline during 3 years of odanacatib and 2 years of odanacatib and 1 year of placebo. (*From* Eisman J, Bone HG, Hosking DJ, et al. Odanacatib in the treatment of post-menopausal women with low bone mineral density: three-year continued therapy and resolution of effect. J Bone Miner Res 2011;26:247; with permission.)

mechanism, but may be the result of fasting or food intake. Glucagonlike peptide 2 (GLP-2) is a polypeptide released from the intestinal mucosa after food intake. Treatment with GLP-2 at bedtime results in a significant reduction in bone resorption that normally occurs overnight. GLP-2 does not reduce bone formation, as shown by osteocalcin levels. A 120-day phase 2 trial in 160 postmenopausal women given GLP-2 resulted in an increase in hip bone density, a reduction in the nocturnal increase in carboxy-terminal collagen crosslinks with no effect on osteocalcin.[16,17] If this pattern were sustained, GLP-2 would have an advantage compared with available antiresorptive agents that decrease bone formation.

Nitrates

Both the Study of Osteoporotic Fractures (SOF) and the Canadian Multicenter Osteoporosis Study (CaMOS) showed small increases in bone mass and reduction in fractures in nitrate users.[18–20] In animals and humans, increases in markers of bone formation and decreases in markers of bone resorption have been shown with nitrate therapy.[21–23] A case control study in Denmark reported a 15% reduction in hip fractures in patients on nitrates.[24] The NOVEL trial (Nitroglycerine as an Option: Value in Early Bone Loss), a 3-year RCT that compared placebo with nitrates in early postmenopausal women, showed no bone mineral density (BMD) increase.[25] A 24-month RCT trial of once daily nitroglycerine (NTG) ointment, 15 mg/d given at night, versus placebo enrolled 243 women with BMD with a T-score between 0 and −2.0.[26] Compared with placebo, subjects on NTG had increases in BMD ($P = .001$) in the lumbar spine (6.7%), femoral neck (7.0%), and total hip (6.2%) at 24 months (**Fig. 6**). NTG significantly ($P<.05$) increased trabecular density (11.9%), cortical density (2.2%), cortical area (10.6%), cortical thickness (13.9%), periosteal circumference (7.4%), polar moment of inertia (7.3%), and polar section modulus (10.7%). Markers of bone resorption (NTx) declined, whereas a marker of bone formation (bone-specific alkaline phosphatase) increased (**Fig. 7**). This uncoupling of bone remodeling is unlike typical antiresorptive agents. Headache was the most common side effect. This drug is inexpensive and further evaluations are ongoing.

ANABOLIC AGENTS

Anabolic agents increase bone mass to a greater degree than antiresorptive agents. These agents are not only able to increase bone mass but also to improve bone quality and increase bone strength, in part by affecting microarchitectural features, such as connectivity density, and geometric features such as diameter. Recombinant human PTH_{1-34}, teriparatide, is the only anabolic agent currently available in the United States. Recombinant human PTH_{1-84} is available in Europe for the treatment of patients with LBM.[27] In patients treated with PTH therapy, bone density changes are underestimated by dual X-ray absorptiometry. When quantitative CT, a volumetric measure of bone mass, is used to measure change in bone density during PTH treatment, increases are significantly greater than with dual X-ray absorptiometry, an areal measure of bone mass.[28] Because the use of PTH is limited to 2 years in the United States and 18 months in Europe, there is an unmet need for additional anabolic agents.

Wnt Signaling: Sclerostin and Dickkopf-1

The discovery and elucidation of the underlying causes of HBM and LBM phenotypes in humans have resulted in many potential drug targets for osteoporosis therapy. Wnt proteins are a large family of extracellular cysteine-rich glycoproteins that help

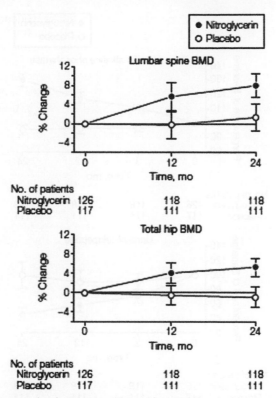

Fig. 6. Percent change in lumbar spine and total hip BMD by dual-energy X-ray absorptiometry over 2 years in subjects treated with nitroglycerin or placebo. (*From* Jamal SA, Hamilton CJ, Eastell R, et al. Effect of nitroglycerin ointment on bone density and strength in postmenopausal women: a randomized trial. JAMA 2011;305:803; with permission.)

regulate embryogenetic bone remodeling and are involved in many additional cellular processes.[29,30] Wnt proteins activate an intracellular pathway that results in accumulation of B-catenin. Wnt allows association of the membrane receptors frizzled and lipoprotein receptor-related protein 5/6, and activation of a protein complex consisting of axin, adenomatous polyposis coli, and glycogen synthase kinase 3, activating an intracellular pathway (**Fig. 8**). In the absence of Wnt, glycogen synthase kinase 3 phosphorylates B-catenin, which is then degraded via the ubiquitin/proteosome pathway. In the presence of Wnt, the protein complex is disrupted and phosphorylation does not occur, B-catenin accumulates, translocates to the cell nucleus, and binds to transcription factors that affect gene transcription, which are important in bone formation.

Inhibitors of Wnt signaling bind to frizzled (serum frizzled–related proteins), Wnt (Wnt inhibitory factors), or lipoprotein receptor–related protein 5/6 (sclerostin and Dickkopf-1). These agonist proteins prevent Wnt from activating the frizzled–lipoprotein receptor–related protein 5/6 receptor signaling pathway, leading to a decrease in signaling and a consequent decrease in bone formation. By contrast, deficiencies in these inhibitors or antibodies to the inhibitors result in increased Wnt signaling and, therefore, increased bone formation.

A human disease of HBM, sclerosteosis, is the result of a homozygous mutation in the *SOST* gene, which encodes sclerostin.[31] A deficiency of sclerostin results in

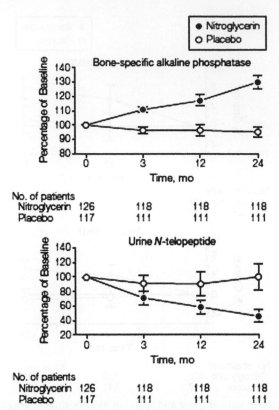

Fig. 7. Percent change in bone-specific alkaline phosphatase (marker of bone formation) and urine N-telopeptide over 2 years in subjects treated with nitroglycerin or placebo. (*From* Jamal SA, Hamilton CJ, Eastell R, et al. Effect of nitroglycerin ointment on bone density and strength in postmenopausal women: a randomized trial. JAMA 2011;305:805; with permission.)

increased Wnt signaling and high bone mass, and in the skull results in entrapment of cranial nerves, increased intracranial pressure, and can subsequently lead to stroke. Heterozygous mutations in the *SOST* gene result in moderate increases in bone mass and fewer skeletal complications. Because sclerostin is a protein that is almost exclusively a product of osteocytes, antibodies offer a way to specifically target bone formation. Antibodies to sclerostin increase bone formation in osteopenic estrogen-deficient rats. A single subcutaneous dose of an antibody to sclerostin in postmenopausal women resulted in an increase in N-terminal propeptide of type I collagen levels of 60% to 100% at day 84 of treatment, no increase in serum *C*-telopeptides, and a 6% increase in lumbar spine bone density.[32]

Osteoporosis pseudoglioma (OPPG), a syndrome associated with LBM and blindness, is caused by an inactivating mutation in LRP5 that inhibits Lrp5-frizzled binding, whereas an HBM phenotype is caused by a point mutation in Lrp5 (G171V).[33] The G171V mutation inhibits the ability of Dkk1, an inhibitor of Wnt signaling, to bind to LRP5. These syndromes show the central role of LRP5 in regulation of bone mass. Gain-of-function mutations in the gene encoding lipoprotein receptor–related protein 5/6 lead to increased bone mass. These mutations impair binding of Dkk1 to LRP5/6

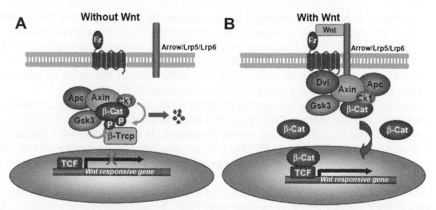

Fig. 8. Simplified view or Wnt/ß-catenin signaling. (*A*) Without Wnt, the scaffolding protein Axin assembles a protein complex, ß-catenin is phosphorylated, ubiquitinated, and degraded by the proteosome. (*B*) With Wnt, ß-catenin is not phosphorylated and is translocated to the nucleus, where it binds to the TCF transcription factor activating Wnt-responsive genes. This signaling cascade is initiated by the Wnt-induced Fz-LRP5/6 coreceptor complex. Apc, antigen presenting cell; ß-cat, ß-catenin; Ck1, casein kinase 1; Dvl, disheveled; GsK3, glycogen synthase kinase 3; LRP, lipoprotein receptor–related protein; TCF, T-cell factor.

and allow increased Wnt signaling and bone formation. Dkk1 antibodies prevent binding of Dickkopf-1 to lipoprotein receptor–related protein 5/6 and increase bone mass, volume, and formation in rodents. Antibodies to Dickkopf-1 could also be used in an anabolic agent for the treatment of patients with LBM.

Serotonin

It has been assumed that the abnormalities in Wnt signaling that result in the HBM and LBM phenotypes described earlier are the result of abnormal signaling in osteoblast and osteocytes. New data suggest that the homeostatic function of LRP5 and Wnt signaling may reside not in the bone but in the enterochromaffin (EC) cells of the duodenum and serotonergic receptors in the brain. Lipoprotein receptor–related protein (LRP) receptors on EC cells regulate synthesis and secretion of peripheral serotonin (gut-derived serotonin [GDS]). GDS accounts for 95% of total serotonin and its production is controlled by the rate-limiting enzyme tryptophan hydroxylase 1 (Tph 1). Outside the brain, a decrease in serotonin favors an increase in osteoblast function. Decreasing serotonin levels normalizes bone formation and bone mass in LRP5-deficient mice. Serotonin inhibits osteoblast proliferation by binding the 5-hydroxytryptamine receptor 1B (Htr1b) on osteoblast membranes.

Yadav and colleagues[34] in a series of experiments showed that targeted deletion of LRP5 in osteoblasts failed to cause osteopenia in mice, suggesting that the signaling pathways involving Lrp5 are indirect and do not reside in osteoblasts. Targeted G171V mutation in osteoblasts in mice did not reproduce the HBM phenotype seen in humans with this mutation, suggesting again that LRP5 signaling does not reside in osteoblasts. Global deletion of LRP5 in all tissues causes increased levels of Tph1, the rate-limiting enzyme in serotonin synthesis outside the brain, and results in increased serotonin levels and decreased osteoblast function. Mice with global LRP5 G171V mutation have low serotonin levels and HBM. Targeted deletion of LRP5 in EC cells in the gut, the source of 95% of all serotonin produced in the body, results in an

LBM phenotype. An HBM phenotype is reproduced by knocking-in the G171 LRP5 mutant in EC cells but not in osteoblasts. Preliminary data on a small number of patients with OPPG show increased serotonin levels, whereas patients with HBM have low serotonin levels. The investigators conclude that the effect of LRP5 binding abnormalities seen in patients with OPPG and HBM are not the result of abnormal signaling in osteoblasts but a result of LRP5 effects on GDS.

Manipulation of GDS may be possible and may have an anabolic effect. LP533401 is a small molecule that inhibits Tph1, the initial enzyme in GDS synthesis. LP533401 is an investigational drug for irritable bowel syndrome. In mice, LP533401 decreases serotonin levels. The effect of LP533401 in an ovariectomized mouse model was equivalent to the effect of PTH on bone mass, indicating that the reduction in serotonin levels had a significant anabolic effect.

Although only 5% of serotonin is produced in the brain, it seems that brain-derived serotonin (BDS) is dominant, compared with GDS, in regulating bone turnover. The brainstem is the principle site of synthesis of tryptophan hydroxylase 2 (Tph2), which is essential for serotonin synthesis in the brain. Global deletion of Tph2 results in an LBM phenotype that is a result of both decreased bone formation and increased bone resorption. Unlike the effect of serotonin in the periphery, which affects only bone formation, central serotonin affects both formation and resorption. This LBM phenotype occurred even when Tph1 outside the brain was also deleted (the Tph1 deletion alone would result in low peripheral serotonin and an HBM phenotype). The LBM phenotype could be rescued when mice were made with heterozygous or homozygous deletion of the gene in central nervous system tissues encoding the B_2 adrenergic receptor, which results in reduced sympathetic tone. Because serotonin does not cross the blood-brain barrier, the sympathetic nervous system is the pathway by which alterations in BDS affect bone turnover. Serotonin uptake reinhibitors (SSRIs) have been associated with lower bone mass and increased risk of fracture.[35]

A central tenet of bone biology has been that sex steroids are the principal modulators of bone remodeling. Ob/ob mice have mutations in the gene for the protein hormone leptin and are obese and have HBM. Ducy and colleagues[36] observed that ob/ob mice that lacked gonadal steroids had HBM. This skeletal phenotype was the result of the loss of leptin signaling in the hypothalamus. Leptin is an adipocyte-derived hormone that regulates a wide range of homeostatic functions by binding to its receptor, ObRb, present in the central nervous system. This model showed that central control was predominant compared with gonadal steroids in bone remodeling. The central control of bone remodeling is mediated by sympathetic tone from the brain through the B_2 adrenergic receptor expressed in osteoblasts. Leptin plays a central role in the regulation of bone mass by activation of specific leptin receptors (ObRb) present in the ventromedial hypothalamus, which reduces serotonin synthesis and firing of serotonergic neurons. Serotonin in the brain favors bone mass accrual.[37,38] The potential for targeting this network pharmacologically is significant, both in the brain and gut.

Calcium-sensing Receptor

The calcium-sensing receptor (CaSR) is a G protein–coupled, 7-pass transmembrane molecule present in the parathyroid gland (and kidney) that functions to monitor and control calcium homeostasis by releasing PTH.[39] Manipulation of the receptor by small-molecule allosteric modulators can affect PTH secretion. Positive allosteric modulators (agonists, calcimimetics) are used to lower PTH secretion in patients with renal disease and hyperparathyroidism (cinacalcet). Negative allosteric modulators (antagonists, calcilytics) are in development and block receptor function resulting in

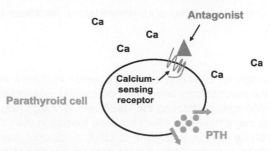

Fig. 9. The effect of a CaSR antagonist on the parathyroid cell. Engagement of the receptor by the antagonist results in release of PTH from the parathyroid cell.

a PTH pulse with each dose (**Fig. 9**). These agents can be given orally and do not require daily injections as with teriparatide. There are several important features of calcilytics that are required to make them useful anabolic agents. They must stimulate the release of sufficient PTH to be anabolic. Anabolic action requires a short T1/2 and transient activation of the receptor because prolonged activation results in prolonged PTH secretion and a catabolic state like hyperparathyroidism. The molecule should not exhaust the parathyroid gland, and not result in hyperplasia. A proof-of-concept study with a calcilytic, SB-751689, (ronacaleret), has shown a robust PTH response, short T1/2, increases in both cortical and trabecular bone formation in animals, and significant (equivalent to teriparatide) increases in markers of osteoblast function (P1NP, osteocalcin, and bone specific alkaline phosphatase [BSAP]). However, a recent dose-ranging clinical trial in humans was discontinued because of poor BMD response.

PTH-related Protein

PTH-related protein (PTHrP) and PTH are related molecules that stimulate the PTH/PTHrP receptor. PTHrP was identified as the cause of humoral hypercalcemia of malignancy (HHM), a severe syndrome in which tumors secreted PTHrP. PTHrP was found to be a ubiquitous local paracrine and autocrine factor produced by most tissues. Mice with heterozygous gene deletion for PTHrP (PTHrP±) have a significant reduction in bone mass; mice with homozygous gene deletion for PTH (PTH−/−) have increased bone mass.[40] As with intermittent injections of PTH, injections of PTHrP are associated with an anabolic response in humans; however, unlike PTH, PTHrP is not associated with activation of osteoclasts and hypercalcemia. Clinical studies of PTHrP have shown it to be less calcemic with markedly lower increases in $1,25(OH)_2D$ than PTH. A 3-month trial of PTHrP (1–36) 400 μg daily as a subcutaneous injection in 16 postmenopausal women with osteoporosis resulted in a 4.7% increase on lumbar spine BMD, and increase in a marker of bone formation (osteocalcin), but no increase in markers of bone resorption (N-telopeptide or deoxypyridinoline), and no hypercalcemia.[41] A subsequent study in 41 healthy postmenopausal women given escalating doses of PTHrP (1–36) up to 750 μg/d revealed no increase in markers of bone resorption with only mild calcemic effects.[42] Thus, PTHrP displays features suggesting that it may be a pure anabolic agent, unlike PTH, which is a mixed anabolic/catabolic agent. This finding makes PTHrP an attractive agent for treatment of severe osteoporosis. BA058, a PTHrP preparation, is currently recruiting for a phase 3 randomized trail comparing placebo, BA058, and teriparatide (n = 2400) with a primary outcome measure of new vertebral fractures, and secondary outcome measure of BMD, hypercalcemia, and nonvertebral fractures over 18 months (ClinicalTrials.gov).

SUMMARY

Advances in the therapy for LBM may soon be possible and are a result of increased understanding of the mechanisms underlying osteoblast, osteoclast, and osteocyte biology. New anabolic agents affecting the CaSR and Wnt signaling, and new antiresorptive agents that might have less effect on bone formation than currently available therapies, offer promise for the treatment of LBM. Additional therapies, especially those that treat patients with established fractures, are needed to reduce the burden of this disease.

REFERENCES

1. Kogianni G, Noble BS. The biology of osteocytes. Curr Osteoporos Rep 2007;5:81–6.
2. Bonewald LF. The amazing osteocyte. J Bone Miner Res 2011;26(2):229–38.
3. Khosla S, Westendorf JJ, Oursler MJ. Building bone to reverse osteoporosis and repair fractures. J Clin Invest 2008;118:421–8.
4. Vahle JL, Sato M, Long GG, et al. Skeletal changes in rats given daily subcutaneous injections of recombinant human parathyroid hormone (1–34) for 2 years and relevance to human safety. Toxicol Pathol 2002;30:312–21.
5. Subbiah V, Madsen VS, Raymond AK, et al. Of mice and men: divergent risks of teriparatide-induced osteosarcoma. Osteoporos Int 2010;21:1041–5.
6. Russell RG, Xia Z, Dunford JE, et al. Bisphosphonates: an update on mechanisms of action and how these relate to clinical efficacy. Ann N Y Acad Sci 2007;1117:209–57.
7. Del Fattore A, Peruzzi B, Rucci N, et al. Clinical, genetic, and cellular analysis of 49 osteopetrotic patients: implications for diagnosis and treatment. J Med Genet 2006;43:315–25.
8. Vasiljeva O, Reinheckel T, Peters C, et al. Emerging roles of cysteine cathepsins in disease and their potential as drug targets. Curr Pharm Des 2007;13:387–403.
9. Stoch SA, Wagner JA. Cathepsin K inhibitors: a novel target for osteoporosis therapy. Clin Pharmacol Ther 2008;83:172–6.
10. Gelb BD, Shi GP, Chapman HA, et al. Pycnodysostosis, a lysosomal disease caused by cathepsin K deficiency. Science 1996;273:1236–8.
11. Gauthier JY, Chauret N, Cromlish W, et al. The discovery of odanacatib (MK-0822), a selective inhibitor of cathepsin K. Bioorg Med Chem Lett 2008;18:923–8.
12. Bone HG, McClung MR, Roux C, et al. Odanacatib, a cathepsin-K inhibitor for osteoporosis: a two-year study in postmenopausal women with low bone density. J Bone Miner Res 2010;25(5):937–47.
13. Eisman JA, Bone HG, Hosking DJ, et al. Odanacatib in the treatment of postmenopausal women with low bone mineral density: three-year continued therapy and resolution of effect. J Bone Miner Res 2011;26:242–51.
14. Bauer DC. Discontinuation of odanacatib and other osteoporosis treatments: here today and gone tomorrow? J Bone Miner Res 2011;26:239–41.
15. Henriksen DB, Alexandersen P, Hartmann B, et al. Disassociation of bone resorption and formation by GLP-2: a 14-day study in healthy postmenopausal women. Bone 2007;40:723–9.
16. Henriksen DB, Alexandersen P, Hartmann B, et al. GLP-2 significantly increases hip BMD in postmenopausal women: a 120-day study. J Bone Miner Res 2007; 22(Suppl 1):S37.

17. Henriksen DB, Alexandersen P, Hartmann B, et al. GLP-2 acutely uncouples bone resorption and bone formation in postmenopausal women. J Bone Miner Res 2008;23:S474.
18. Jamal S, Hamilton C, Black D, et al. Nitroglycerine improves bone mineral density, bone geometry, and bone strength: results from a two-year randomized controlled trial. J Bone Miner Res 2010;25:S77.
19. Jamal SA, Cummings SR, Hawker GA. Isosorbide mononitrate increases bone formation and decreases bone resorption in postmenopausal women: a randomized trial. J Bone Miner Res 2004;19:1512–7.
20. Cummings SR, Browner WS, Bauer D, et al. Endogenous hormones and the risk of hip and vertebral fractures among older women. Study of Osteoporotic Fractures Research Group. N Engl J Med 1998;339:733–8.
21. Wimalawansa SJ. Nitric oxide and bone. Ann N Y Acad Sci 2010;1192:391–403.
22. Wimalawansa SJ. Nitric oxide: new evidence for novel therapeutic indications. Expert Opin Pharmacother 2008;9:1935–54.
23. Wimalawansa SJ. Rationale for using nitric oxide donor therapy for prevention of bone loss and treatment of osteoporosis in humans. Ann N Y Acad Sci 2007; 1117:283–97.
24. Pouwels S, Lalmohamed A, van Staa T, et al. Use of organic nitrates and the risk of hip fracture: a population-based case-control study. J Clin Endocrinol Metab 2010;95:1924–31.
25. Wimalawansa SJ, Grimes JP, Wilson AC, et al. Transdermal nitroglycerin therapy may not prevent early postmenopausal bone loss. J Clin Endocrinol Metab 2009; 94:3356–64.
26. Jamal SA, Hamilton CJ, Eastell R, et al. Effect of nitroglycerin ointment on bone density and strength in postmenopausal women: a randomized trial. JAMA 2011;305:800–7.
27. Neer RM, Arnaud CD, Zanchetta JR, et al. Effect of parathyroid hormone (1–34) on fractures and bone mineral density in postmenopausal women with osteoporosis. N Engl J Med 2001;344:1434–41.
28. McClung MR, San Martin J, Miller PD, et al. Opposite bone remodeling effects of teriparatide and alendronate in increasing bone mass. Arch Intern Med 2005;165: 1762–8.
29. Glass DA 2nd, Karsenty G. In vivo analysis of Wnt signaling in bone. Endocrinology 2007;148:2630–4.
30. Baron R, Rawadi G. Targeting the Wnt/beta-catenin pathway to regulate bone formation in the adult skeleton. Endocrinology 2007;148:2635–43.
31. Gardner JC, van Bezooijen RL, Mervis B, et al. Bone mineral density in sclerosteosis; affected individuals and gene carriers. J Clin Endocrinol Metab 2005; 90:6392–5.
32. Padhi D, Stouch B, Fang L, et al. Anti-sclerostin antibody increases markers of bone formation in healthy postmenopausal women. J Bone Miner Metab 2007; 22(Suppl 1):S37.
33. Williams BO, Insogna KL. Where Wnts went: the exploding field of Lrp5 and Lrp6 signaling in bone. J Bone Miner Res 2009;24:171–8.
34. Yadav VK, Balaji S, Suresh PS, et al. Pharmacological inhibition of gut-derived serotonin synthesis is a potential bone anabolic treatment for osteoporosis. Nat Med 2010;16:308–12.
35. Richards JB, Papaioannou A, Adachi JD, et al. Effect of selective serotonin reuptake inhibitors on the risk of fracture. Arch Intern Med 2007;167:188–94.

36. Ducy P, Amling M, Takeda S, et al. Leptin inhibits bone formation through a hypothalamic relay: a central control of bone mass. Cell 2000;100:197–207.
37. Rosen CJ. Bone: serotonin, leptin and the central control of bone remodeling. Nat Rev Rheumatol 2009;5:657–8.
38. Rosen CJ. Serotonin rising–the bone, brain, bowel connection. N Engl J Med 2009;360:957–9.
39. Brown EM. The calcium-sensing receptor: physiology, pathophysiology and CaR-based therapeutics. Subcell Biochem 2007;45:139–67.
40. Amizuka N, Karaplis AC, Luz A, et al. Haploinsufficiency of parathyroid hormone-related peptide results in abnormal postnatal bone development. Dev Biol 1996; 175:166–76.
41. Horwitz MJ, Tedesco B, Gundberg C, et al. Short-term parathyroid hormone-related protein as a skeletal anabolic agent for the treatment of postmenopausal osteoporosis. J Clin Endocrinol Metab 2003;88:569–75.
42. Horwitz MJ, Tedesco B, Garcia-Ocana A, et al. Parathyroid hormone-related protein for the treatment of postmenopausal osteoporosis: defining the maximal tolerable dose. J Clin Endocrinol Metab 2010;95(3):1279–87.

Calcium and Vitamin D Controversies

David S. Silver, MD[a,b,*]

KEYWORDS

• Calcium • Vitamin D • Osteoporosis • Controversy

Calcium and vitamin D have been cornerstones for prevention and treatment of osteoporosis for decades. Even before clear and convincing evidence of their efficacy, the use of both calcium and vitamin D was routinely recommended by physicians, most specifically in postmenopausal women, to maintain bone health. However, in the last 10 years, there has been increased interest in the role of vitamin D in preventing or treating a wide range of diseases, including cancer, diabetes, autoimmune disease, and cardiovascular disease. Testing for vitamin D levels has become more common and practitioners are often recommending high doses of vitamin D, with limited clinical data to support them. In addition, recent data have suggested that calcium, which had always been assumed to be safe, may have a role in increasing the risk of cardiovascular disease. Further, new types of calcium have been introduced into the market claiming to have improved absorption and tolerability, with little if any scientific evidence to support these claims. This article examines some of the controversies pertaining to calcium and vitamin D, both the reported benefits and potential harms that have been reported.

DOSING

There has been great debate about the proper level of intake of calcium and vitamin D, based on the significant amount of conflicting data that exists in the literature. Much of this is the result of data that suggest that vitamin D intake may have significant health benefits including reduction in cancer, prevention of autoimmunity including diabetes, prevention of preeclampsia in pregnancy, and decreases in heart attack and strokes. When evaluating the issue of appropriate levels of calcium and vitamin D intake, one must review the existing data for skeletal manifestations and complications of low vitamin D or calcium intake (or high intake) versus the extraskeletal potential benefits or risks that have been raised. Therefore, this article separates these 2 issues of skeletal health versus extraskeletal health as they relate to appropriate levels of calcium and vitamin D intake, and examines the potential complications and benefits that could be realized.

No funding support, disclosures, or conflicts to report.
[a] Cedars-Sinai Medical Center/UCLA School of Medicine, Los Angeles, CA, USA
[b] OMC Clinical Research Center, 8641 Wilshire Boulevard, Suite 301, Beverly Hills, CA 90211, USA
* OMC Clinical Research Center, 8641 Wilshire Boulevard, Suite 301, Beverly Hills, CA 90211.
E-mail address: davids@OMCresearch.org

Both calcium and vitamin D are necessary for normal bone formation. Calcium is a major constituent of bone matrix, and vitamin D is necessary for intestinal absorption of calcium and uptake into bone. Vitamin D can be produced in the skin; however, even in warm-weather climates, people often produce inadequate vitamin D and require exogenous sources as supplementation.[1-3] Vitamin D, along with parathyroid hormone and calcitonin, play an integral role in calcium and phosphorus metabolism in target tissues, specifically bone, intestine, and kidney. Vitamin D must be metaboli-cally activated before having a physiologic effect (**Fig. 1**).[4] 7-Dehydrocholesterol is photometabolized in the skin to vitamin D_3, and then undergoes 25-hydroxylation in the liver. The 25-hydroxyvitamin D_3 is further hydroxylated to 1,25-dihydroxyvitamin D_3, which is the most biologically active form, or to 24,25-dihydroxyvitamin D_3. The kidney regulates how much of the active form (ie, 1,25-dihydroxyvitamin D_3) is avail-able, based on serum calcium levels.

In addition, when vitamin D levels are low, patients can develop secondary hyper-parathyroidism. When vitamin D levels are low, parathyroid hormone is secreted to raise serum calcium levels, causing increasing bone resorption and normalization of calcium activity, and therefore vitamin D deficiency secondary to hyperparathyroidism may result in significant bone loss and increased fracture risk. Adequate supplemen-tation with vitamin D can reduce or eliminate the secondary hyperparathyroidism, and reduce the fracture risk. Usually a 25-OH vitamin level of 30 µg/dL is necessary to elim-inate secondary hyperparathyroidism.[5,6] When vitamin D levels are adequate, calcium

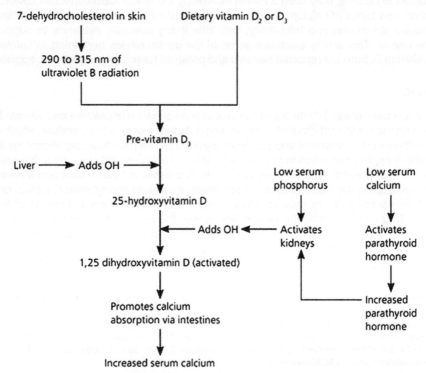

Fig. 1. Metabolic activation of vitamin D. (*Adapted from* Bordelon P, Ghetu M, Langan R. Recognition and management of vitamin D deficiency. Am Fam Physician 2009;80:841–6; with permission.)

absorption from the intestinal tract averages about 30% to 40%. In vitamin D–deficient states, calcium absorption decreases to about 10% to 15%. To maintain serum calcium levels, parathyroid hormone is released, secondary hyperparathyroidism occurs, and calcium is released from bone.

Supplementation with vitamin D_3 (cholecalciferol) is more effective than vitamin D_2, and therefore is the preferred mode of supplementation. As stated earlier, calcium homeostasis is regulated through numerous hormones, most specifically 1,25-dihydroxyvitamin D_3, and it is required for normal bone homeostasis. Maintenance of serum calcium levels is the primary function of these regulatory hormones, so if serum calcium, in response to either hypercalciuria, inadequate intake, or other mechanisms, is noted, the body will attempt to regulate these hormones. Inadequate intake of calcium has been associated with lower bone mineral densities.[7]

Supplementation of calcium and vitamin D_3 at the previous Recommended Daily Allowance, although showing increase in bone density, has not consistently been associated with decreased fracture rates in population analyses. Supplementation with calcium 1000 mg per day and vitamin D_3 400 international units (IU) per day, although associated with increased hip bone mineral density, has not been not associated with a statistically significant reduction in fractures.[8]

However, some studies have shown that patients taking calcium and vitamin D do have a reduction in overall fracture risk, although the mechanism may be independent of its skeletal effects. Numerous studies have shown that adequate vitamin D is important in fall prevention.[9–13] Vitamin D receptors are prevalent in muscle cells, and several vitamin D receptors on muscle cells decrease with age. By binding to the receptors on muscle cells, several pathways are activated, which allows calcium uptake in the muscle cells. In addition, phosphate metabolism increases and muscle cell proliferation or differentiation occurs. 1,25-Dihydroxyvitamin D may also modulate muscle contractility. Patients with significant vitamin D deficiency have type 2 fiber atrophy of the muscles. Numerous studies have shown that patients who received vitamin D supplementation, be it vitamin D_3, vitamin D_2, or even activated vitamin D supplements, were shown to have decreased risk of falling when given in concentrations of greater than 700 IU per day. However, megadosing of vitamin D_3 administered yearly at 500,000 IU resulted in increased fall rates within the first 3 months of supplementation and increased fracture,[14] suggesting that daily therapy may be preferred to large doses given less frequently.

Reduced risk of falling likely translates into reduced risk of fractures, specifically hip fracture, especially when serum concentrations of vitamin D are increased. These effects likely become more important as patients get older, because low vitamin D levels are more prevalent and there are decreased numbers of vitamin D receptors on muscle cells. Therefore, if vitamin D and calcium reduce fractures, it is possible that the mechanism may be independent of changes in bone density, but may also be related to increased muscle strength and reduction in fall risk.

Although few would dispute the need for supplementation of calcium and vitamin D_3, there is a paucity of randomized, controlled data examining this question. Studies typically involve retrospective analyses, and cannot control for dietary intake, sun exposure, or even use of supplements. In 2010, the Institute of Medicine attempted to review the dietary reference intakes based on the best data available.[15–17] Although most studies are of levels of supplementation of calcium in the range from 500 to 1000 mg per day, and of vitamin D_3 in the range from 400 to 1000 units per day, many investigators have suggested that higher-dose supplementation of vitamin D may provide additional benefits. However, there are few, if any, consistent data for very high-dose vitamin D intake (>10,000 IU/d), and oversupplementation may have potential side effects. Ingestion of too much calcium or vitamin D may have its own set of issues as well. Many patients may be intolerant of certain calcium preparations. Increased consumption of calcium has been associated with hypercalciuria and nephrolithiasis, and concerns have been raised regarding cardiovascular complications, specifically vascular calcification (discussed later), constipation, and interaction with the absorption of other minerals. High levels of vitamin D have been associated with increased risk of fracture, when getting more than 75 µg per deciliter. Other concerns regarding vitamin D include increased risk of mortality (eg, from pancreatic cancer), potential cardiovascular risk related to increased hypercalcemia and hypercalciuria, as well as growth retardation in children and infants. Therefore, recommendations about use of high-dose vitamin D at this time, without adequate substantiation in the literature, cannot be recommended.

However, the old recommendation of 400 units of vitamin D seems not to have been adequate. The Institute of Medicine based recommendations on the Recommended Daily Allowance, which is derived from the Estimated Average Requirement (EAR) and needs to exceed the requirement for 97.5% of the population. The EAR represents the estimated median requirement, necessary for adequate need for 50% of the population.

When taking into account these recommendations, the dietary intake of calcium and degree of sun exposure are difficult to quantify and may affect a patient's individual need. In addition, upper limits of tolerability may be present, more than which there is increased risk to certain individuals, and therefore the Institute of Medicine developed tolerable upper intake level (UL), which is the average high daily intake that is likely to pose no risk of adverse events to any individual in the population. For most patients, dietary calcium recommended intake ranges from 1000 to 1300 mg per day, although, after menopause, calcium requirements slightly increase (**Table 1**). This intake is contradictory to some earlier recommendations of 1500 mg per day that were advanced by certain organizations. In addition, it is important to emphasize that not all calcium supplementation should be taken at once, because it may overwhelm the intestine's ability to absorb, so it must be done in split dosing, not to exceed 500 to 600 mg per dose.

The dietary intake for vitamin D is more controversial, because recommendations have varied from as low as 400 IU per day of vitamin D_3 to as high as 2000 to 4000 IU per day, depending on the perspective of the author and interpretation of the literature. However, there is little debate in the literature that increasing to at least 600 to 800 IU per day is safe and may provide additional benefits, although there are patients who may benefit from greater amounts, based on certain individual disease conditions.[18] Many would argue that at least 1000 IU of vitamin D_3 per day, or 2000 IU per day if there is evidence of vitamin D deficiency, would be appropriate, with the goal of achieving a 25-OH vitamin D level of 30 ng/dL.[19] The advocates of high-dose vitamin D_3 also must remember the potential complications that have been found in numerous studies. Therefore, the upper limit of tolerability was established for men and women, increasing it to 4000 IU, although the report suggests that up to 10,000 IU per day are probably safe in most circumstances. Although there are those who advocate use of higher doses, there is little if any support in the literature for this, and there is potential for significant toxicity if advocated on a consistent basis.

There are individual circumstances that require higher doses of calcium and vitamin D. In addition, the role of serum measurement of 25-hydroxyvitamin D has been studied. There are many who advocate routine screening as part of health physicals in an attempt to monitor intake as well as effectiveness and adequate absorption. The prevalence of vitamin D insufficiency is high, and serum measurement can help

Table 1
Dietary reference intakes for calcium and vitamin D

Life Stage Group	Calcium			Vitamin D		
	EAR (mg/d)	Recommended Dietary Allowance (mg/d)	Upper Intake Level (mg/d)	EAR (IU/d)	Recommended Dietary Allowance (IU/d)	Upper Intake Level (IU/d)
Infants 0–6 mo	a	a	1000	b	b	1000
Infants 6–12 mo	a	a	1500	b	—	1500
1–3 y	500	700	2500	400	600	2500
4–8 y	800	1000	2500	400	600	3000
9–13 y	1100	1300	3000	400	600	4000
14–18 y	1100	1300	3000	400	600	4000
19–30 y	800	1000	2500	400	600	4000
31–50 y	800	1000	2500	400	600	4000
51–70 y (men)	800	1000	2000	400	600	4000
51–70 y (women)	1000	1200	2000	400	600	4000
>70 y	1000	1200	2000	400	800	4000
14–18 y (pregnant/lactating)	1100	1300	3000	400	600	4000
19–50 y (pregnant/lactating)	800	1000	2500	400	600	4000

[a] For infants, adequate intake is 200 mg/d for 0 to 6 months of age and 260 mg/d for 6 to 12 months of age.
[b] For infants, adequate intake is 400 IU/d for 0 to 6 months of age and 400 IU/d for 6 to 12 months of age.

to solve this. However, this may present an undue economic burden and, in lower-risk populations, this may not be considered cost-effective.

A level of greater than 20 ng/dL is considered necessary for maintenance of bone health, although many believe that a level of 30 ng/dL or more might be a better target for the other extraskeletal manifestations. Some studies, including randomized controlled data, suggested that raising 25-hydroxyvitamin D levels from 21 to 29 ng/mL reduces fracture risk by up to 33%.[20] The Institute of Medicine report targets a level of 20 ng/dL, citing a lack of consistency in the literature for benefits at more than that level. Many have been critical of this approach, citing that dosing of 600 IU/d of vitamin D_3 is often inadequate even to assume a level of 20 ng/dL, the lack of side effects when pushing the level to 30 ng/mL, and the literature that does support benefits both for bone and elsewhere. Therefore, supplementation of at least 1000 IU/d seems safe and appropriate in almost any circumstance. Use of a high dose of vitamin D weekly or monthly without adequate screening or in low-risk populations is not indicated based on the best available data and lack of any clear documented benefit compared with daily dosing. No population has been identified in which there is a definite advantage.

Most studies and review articles suggest that the combination of calcium and vitamin D_3 reduces the incidence of fractures in patients with osteoporosis. Studies published by Dawson and colleagues,[21] showed that calcium and vitamin D_3 supplementation did reduce fracture incidence in elderly populations, although it is unclear whether or not this is the sole effect of calcium or of vitamin D. The use of calcium and vitamin D_3 for bone health seems not to be in question at this time.

CALCIUM AND VITAMIN D AND CARDIOVASCULAR RISK

One of the greatest areas of controversy in the literature of late concerns the use of calcium and the increased rate of vascular events. A study published in the British Medical Journal in 2008 concerned 1471 postmenopausal women randomized to receive calcium supplementation or placebo.[22] Patients were followed for 5 years. Myocardial infarctions were more commonly reported in the calcium group than in the placebo group, with $P = .01$, as well as the composite endpoint of myocardial infarction, stroke, or sudden death. Adjudicated myocardial infarctions were at a relative risk of 2.12, and the confidence interval did not overlap 1. However, verified events did not reach statistical significance, even when unreported events were included. Patients were excluded if they had a 25-hydroxyvitamin D level of less than 25 ng/mL. The same researchers from New Zealand performed a meta-analysis of 15 trials, and showed a small but statistically significant increased risk of myocardial infarction, with a hazard ration of 1.31, but did not show statistical significance for any other composite influence including stroke, or combination of myocardial infarction, stroke or sudden death, and death.[23] They concluded that calcium supplements without coadministered vitamin D increase risk of myocardial infarction. These studies were mostly of women (many of the studies were 100% women) and involved a small number of patients, and cardiovascular outcome was not the primary focus.

There have been numerous criticisms that this meta-analysis was flawed. Numerous other studies have drawn different conclusions. For instance, studies by Lappe and Heaney,[24] from the Creighton University database, showed a decrease, although not statistically significant, in myocardial infarctions in patients who were taking calcium supplementation. The Finnish study, which was a prospective observational study, showed an adjusted hazard ratio of 1.24 for coronary heart disease in women who used supplementations; when adjusted for patients who used calcium and calcium with vitamin D, the average was 1.26.[25] Again, this shows a small but statistically significant increase. An observational cohort study from London, by Shah and colleagues,[26] using the UK primary database, which followed 9910 women, showed in the first 2 years after calcium supplementation a numerical, but again not statistically significant, decrease in the number of myocardial infarctions, strokes, or death (hazard ratio 0.82; confidence interval 0.67–1.01).

Animal models have shown varying results as well, although most have shown that calcium supplementation has inhibited atherosclerosis and vascular calcification.[27] Using the Olmstead County (MN) database, a study by Bhakta and colleagues[28] showed that, for aortic valve calcification and coronary artery calcification, there were no statistically significant increases in 4 years.

Studies combining calcium with vitamin D have shown neutral results. In patients in the Women's Health Initiative trial,[29] which had shown overall nonsignificant reduction in overall mortality, a hazard ratio of 0.91 was found, barely missing statistical significance. The patients were assigned to either elemental calcium carbonate 1000 mg per day or vitamin D_3 400 IU per day. In addition, other data from the Women's Health Initiative investigators showed that women taking calcium carbonate at 500 mg with 200 IU of vitamin D twice had no impact on cardiovascular events. It seems that the combination of calcium and vitamin D does not significantly increase or decrease the rate of myocardial infarction.[30] The data for vitamin D supplementation alone seem to suggest a potential benefit, although there is no statistical method that can be accepted as scientifically certain. No randomized trials have been done of this issue. Studies have predominately been retrospective analyses and have not been of a sufficient number or size to draw any reasonable conclusions.

Investigators have theorized potential mechanisms for the possible increase or decrease in cardiovascular events with calcium supplementation, including increase of serum calcium levels by calcium supplementation, which would possibly accelerate vascular calcification. Although calcium supplementation has been associated with beneficial increases of high-density lipoprotein (HDL) cholesterol and reduction of low-density lipoprotein (LDL) cholesterol, it seems that a lipid-related mechanism does not adequately explain the symptoms. Calcium's effect on clotting does not seem to be an issue.

At best, one could conclude that the data are unclear, and not enough to draw any reasonable conclusion, because there is potential for calcium and/or vitamin D to be either causative or protective in the development of coronary artery disease. Meta-analyses of studies that show small changes in risk profile must be interpreted cautiously, because cohort studies and meta-analyses are not intended to detect small changes and therefore may not adequately reflect risk in this population.

VITAMIN D AND CANCER

Much of the recent potential interest in vitamin D research has been related to its possible protective effects in the prevention of cancers. Numerous studies have suggested that lower levels of vitamin D are associated with increased risk of numerous cancers. The more challenging question regards whether vitamin D replacement can either lower the risk of these cancers. Observational studies of pooled analyses have investigated numerous studies of breast cancer, colon cancer, melanoma, ovarian cancer, prostate cancer, and pancreatic cancer. Studies of serum vitamin D levels in patients showed that the lower the vitamin D level, the higher the risk for the development of breast cancer,[31] and that individuals with serum concentrations of 25-hydroxyvitamin D of approximately 52 ng/mL had a 50% lower risk of breast cancer than those with serum 25-hydroxyvitamin D levels of less than 13 ng/mL.[32] Studies in China have also suggested that the highest quintile of circulating 25-hydroxyvitamin D was associated with a 45% decrease in breast cancer compared with the lowest quintile.[33] In addition, there was a 19% decrease in breast cancer in people with the highest quintile of calcium intake compared with the lowest quintile, suggesting that calcium may independently have a protective effect in the development of breast cancer.

Studies of colon cancer progression show risk from the lowest quintile to the highest quintile; patients with a serum 25-hydroxyvitamin D level of greater than or equal to 30 ng/mL had a 50% lower risk of colon cancer compared with patients with a level of less than or equal to 12 ng/mL.[34] Meta-analyses in these populations support the possibility that certain single-nucleotide polymorphisms in the vitamin D receptor may confer a lower risk of breast cancer than in patients who did not have such polymorphisms.[35,36] Similar results were also found in other cancers. However, meta-analyses of patients with ovarian cancer risk and circulating vitamin D found an inverse association, but this did not reach statistical significance.[37] In patients with nonmetastatic prostate cancer, an inverse relationship was again seen, in that vitamin D insufficiency was prevalent among patients with nonmetastatic prostate cancer.[38] Potential mechanisms include vitamin D resulting in transcription of the number of genes involving induction of cell apoptosis and cell-cycle inhibition, therefore attributing to vitamin D antiproliferative and proapoptotic effects on cell lineages. This mechanism may have effects on adaptive immunity as well. It has also been suggested that, in patients with other cancers such as melanoma and pancreatic cancer, the lowest levels of vitamin D have a significantly increased risk of the development of the cancers compared with patients with higher levels of vitamin D,[39,40] although dietary intake of vitamin D may be positively associated with the development of pancreatic cancer.[41]

The more important question may be whether or not this simply represents patients who have poorer nutritional status or poorer health habits, and whether this is simply a marker for these patients, or whether or not correction of vitamin D insufficiency would potentially lead to reduction in cancer risk. There is a paucity of data for this question. Case-controlled studies of patients with breast cancer have suggested such findings,[31] but no high-quality randomized controlled trials, or even prospective trials, of patients taking vitamin D_3 supplementations versus those who are not have been performed to adequately address this issue. Therefore, although giving patients with vitamin D insufficiency supplementation, especially in high-risk populations, seems reasonable, the medical literature cannot yet support supplementation of these patients as a method of prevention of various breast, ovarian, or gastrointestinal (GI) tumors. However, the consistency of data suggests that one may not need to wait until such data become available before deciding to supplement patients. A reasonable position might be that, in patients who are considered high risk, vitamin D screening should be implemented (with the exception of pancreatic cancer), and patients who are found to be insufficient should be treated. A further alternative would be simple supplementation in this high-risk population, within the guidelines presented by the Institute of Medicine, to prevent vitamin D insufficiency (not in excess of 4000 IU/d), in hopes that this might have protective effects against development of these cancers.

VITAMIN D AND AUTOIMMUNE DISEASE

Vitamin D has emerged as a potentially important modulator of autoimmune disease. Vitamin D deficiency has been related to several autoimmune disorders including diabetes, systemic lupus, rheumatoid arthritis, inflammatory bowel disease, and multiple sclerosis (MS).[42] Vitamin D has a significant impact on regulation and differentiating T and B lymphocytes, macrophages, and natural killer cells, and it interferes with the production of certain inflammatory cytokines.[43,44] Reduction in production of proinflammatory cytokines such as interleukin (IL)-2 and tumor necrosis factor α, and inhibition of expression of IL-6 as well as autoantibodies by B lymphocytes, may all be mechanisms by which vitamin D prevents the development of autoimmune disease. In addition, vitamin D has been recognized as having immunomodulating effects. 1,25-Dihydroxyvitamin D has been shown to have immunomodulating effects on T cells, B cells and macrophages, and may help to regulate a switch from Th1 to Th2 regulatory pathways.

Studies implied that patients with low levels of vitamin D may be at increased risk of the development of autoimmune diseases. Rheumatoid arthritis is a predominantly TH1-driven disease, and vitamin D deficiency is associated with exacerbation of a TH1 immune response. Therefore, supplementation with vitamin D may be able to shift the immune response in a way that would reduce antigen-presenting T cells from triggering an immune response. In addition, vitamin D receptor polymorphisms may be linked to increased rheumatoid arthritis susceptibility in patients with vitamin D deficiency.

Observations of patients with lupus have shown that low vitamin D is associated with increases in disease activity.[45] Again, certain polymorphisms in the vitamin D receptor may increase susceptibility to systemic lupus erythematosis.[46,47] Others have theorized that, although low vitamin D levels might not be causative in disease, they may be involved in perpetuating disease symptoms. Patients with reduced vitamin D have been shown to have increased inflammatory cytokine levels and increased production of anti–double-stranded DNA and anti-Smith antigen.[48] However, other studies have not shown the consistency of this variation. Studies have also shown a significant inverse relationship between vitamin D levels and disease activity in patients with established lupus. Some have theorized that these inflammatory mechanisms may also be related to low vitamin D levels in association with heart disease.

Diabetes, now recognized as an autoimmune disease, has also been linked to low serum vitamin D levels. Patients with type 1 and type 2 diabetes have been associated with low vitamin D levels. It has also been well demonstrated that pancreatic tissue, specifically insulin-producing cells in the pancreas, expresses the vitamin D receptor and vitamin D–binding protein, and variations in the genes of the vitamin D receptor may alter vitamin D metabolism, which may alter insulin secretion and inflammation in the pancreas.[49] In addition, plasma calcium levels are involved in regulation of insulin synthesis and secretion, as well as the vitamin D receptor again directly affecting the function of pancreatic β cells. Based on the antiinflammatory and secretory effects, vitamin D deficiency seems to be associated with diabetes. In addition, epidemiologic studies have shown that children who receive daily vitamin D supplementation have a lower risk of developing type 1 diabetes, implying that supplementation of vitamin D can reduce the risk of these problematic diseases. Therefore, one may conclude that, through the antiinflammatory effect by shifting away from TH1-related mechanism may affect inflammation of the pancreas and therefore lead to a lower risk of diabetes mellitus.[50]

Evidence also suggests that low vitamin D levels are associated with increased risk and flare-ups of inflammatory bowel disease and MS. The pathophysiology of inflammatory bowel disease involves Th1 pathways, which are more prevalent in vitamin D–deficient states.[51] Experimental models have shown decreased progression of

MS with vitamin D supplementation and risk of MS may decrease by up to 40% in certain populations who consume high levels of vitamin D.[52]

The data involving vitamin D and autoimmune disease seem to be consistent across numerous disease states, implying that it may have an increasing role in the future in prevention and treatment.

There have also been studies of various other diseases for their potential relationship to low vitamin D and calcium levels. Fibromyalgia has been specifically investigated in small studies, and vitamin D levels were lower in some studies, but not consistently.[53,54]

RECOMMENDATIONS

Based on the best available evidence-based medicine, the Institute of Medicine recommendations for vitamin D seem to be too conservative. As suggested by Heaney[19] and others, a target goal of 30 ng/mL seems to have potential health benefits without any evidence of negative consequences. At least 1000 IU/d of vitamin D_3 would be necessary to maintain this level. In patients who are deemed to be vitamin D deficient, daily dosing of 2000 to 4000 IU vitamin D_3 would be appropriate and safe. Without supportive data, high-dose weekly, monthly, or yearly dosing cannot be recommended at this time. Patients with extremely low vitamin D levels (<10 ng/mL) are at risk for osteomalacia and may require even higher levels of daily supplementation.

Vitamin D screening, specifically 25-OH vitamin D levels, is appropriate in all patients with osteoporosis and other high-risk populations, including those at high risk for falls, malnutrition states such as gastric or intestinal bypass, patients with hepatic or renal disease, those with limited sunlight exposure, patients with chronic musculoskeletal pain, and darker skinned individuals. Screening of others would be considered optional, but only if they are compliant with the dietary recommendations. If data continue to support the protective effects of adequate vitamin D, generalized screening in the population may be reasonable.

Calcium intake as recommended by the Institute of Medicine should be 1000 to 1200 mg/d. Dietary intake, which is preferred to supplementation, should be considered in calculating the need for supplementation, especially in light of concerns raised regarding calcium supplementation and cardiovascular risk. Previous recommendations for 1500 mg/d seem too high. In addition, vitamin D repletion improves calcium absorption, so the lower end of the target goal seems reasonable (1000 mg/d). Calcium citrate, which does not require an acidic environment to be absorbed in the GI tract, is preferred to calcium carbonate, specifically in patients on proton pump inhibitors or in elderly patients who have achlorhydria. With the average American diet including about 300 to 500 mg/d of calcium, supplementation with 500 to 600 mg is often adequate.

SUMMARY

Controversies regarding appropriate use of vitamin D and calcium are predominately related to the extraskeletal effects. Calcium and vitamin D are essential for bone health. The concerns regarding calcium and cardiovascular complications are inconclusive at best, and do not warrant a change in our approach to supplementation at this time. A growing body of literature exists suggesting that additional vitamin D may have numerous benefits, although more study needs to be done. Further prospective trials would provide insight into the potential advantages that increased vitamin D supplementation could provide.

REFERENCES

1. Oren Y, Shapira Y, Agmon-Levin N, et al. Vitamin D insufficiency in a sunny environment: a demographic and seasonal analysis. Isr Med Assoc J 2010;12:751–6.
2. Binkley N, Ramamurthy R, Krueger D. Low vitamin D status: definition, prevalence, consequences, and correction. Endocrinol Metab Clin North Am 2010; 39:287–301.
3. Arabi A, El Rassi R, El-Haji Fuleihan G. Hypovitaminosis D in developing countries-prevalence, risk factors and outcomes. Nat Rev Endocrinol 2010;6:550–61.
4. Bordelon P, Ghetu M, Langan R. Recognition and management of vitamin D deficiency. Am Fam Physician 2009;80:841–6.
5. Thacher T, Clarke B. Vitamin D insufficiency. Mayo Clin Proc 2011;86:50–60.
6. Heaney R. Vitamin D in health and disease. Clin J Am Soc Nephrol 2008;3: 1535–41.
7. Cranney A, Horsley T, O'Donnell S, et al. Effectiveness and safety of vitamin D in relation to bone health. Evid Rep Technol Assess (Full Rep) 2007;(158):1–235.
8. Larrosa M, Gomez A, Casado E, et al. Hypovitaminosis D as a risk factor of hip fracture severity. Osteoporos Int 2011 [Epub ahead of print].
9. Rabenda V, Bruyere O, Reginster J. Relationship between bone mineral density changes and risk of fractures among patients receiving calcium with or without vitamin D supplementation: a meta-regression. Osteoporos Int 2011;22:893–901.
10. Nurmi-Luthje I, Luthje P, Kaukonen J, et al. Post-fracture prescribed calcium and vitamin D supplements alone or, in females, with concomitant anti-osteoporosis drugs is associated with lower mortality in elderly hip fracture patients: a prospective analysis. Drugs Aging 2009;26:409–21.
11. Pfeifer M, Begerow B, Minne H, et al. Effects of a long-term vitamin D and calcium supplementation on falls and parameters of muscle function in community-dwelling older individuals. Osteoporos Int 2009;20:315–22.
12. Bischoff H, Stahelin H, Dick W, et al. Effects of vitamin D and calcium supplementation on falls: a randomized controlled trial. J Bone Miner Res 2003;18:343–51.
13. Bischoff H, Dawson-Hughes B, Orav J, et al. Fall prevention with supplemental and active forms of vitamin D: a meta-analysis of randomized controlled trials. BMJ 2009;339:3692.
14. Sanders K, Stuart S, Williamson E, et al. The efficacy of high-dose oral vitamin D3 administered once a year: a randomized, double-blind, placebo-controlled trial (Vital D study) for fall and fractures in older women. Osteoporos Int 2011; 22(Suppl 1):S104.
15. Dietary reference intakes for calcium and vitamin D. Washington, DC: Institute of Medicine; 2010.
16. Ross A, Manson J, Abrams S, et al. The 2011 report on dietary reference intakes for calcium and vitamin D from the Institute of Medicine: What clinicians need to know. J Clin Endocrinol Metab 2011;96:53–8.
17. Van den Bergh J, Bours S, van Geel T, et al. Optimal use of vitamin D when treating osteoporosis. Curr Osteoporos Rep 2011;9:36–42.
18. Reid I, Avenell I. Evidence-based policy on dietary calcium and vitamin D. J Bone Miner Res 2011;26:452–4.
19. Heaney R, Holick M. Why the IOM recommendations for vitamin D are deficient. J Bone Miner Res 2011;26:455–7.
20. Trivedi D, Doll R, Khaw K. Effect on four monthly oral vitamin D3 (cholecalciferol) supplementation on fractures and mortality in men and women living in the community: a randomized, double-blind, controlled trial. BMJ 2003;236:469–74.

21. Dawson-Hughes B. Serum 25-hydroxyvitamin D and functional outcomes in the elderly. Am J Clin Nutr 2008;88(2):537S–40S.
22. Bolland M, Barber P, Doughty R, et al. Vascular events in healthy older women receiving calcium supplementation: randomized controlled trial. BMJ 2008;336: 262–6.
23. Bolland M, Avenell A, Baron J, et al. Effects of calcium supplements on risk of myocardial infarction and cardiovascular events: meta-analysis. BMJ 2010;341: 3691–9.
24. Lappe J, Heaney R. Results may not be generalisable. BMJ 2008;336:403.
25. Pentti K, Tuppurainen M, Honkanen R, et al. Use of calcium supplements and the risk of coronary heart disease in 52-62-year-old women: the Kuipio Osteoporosis Risk Factor and Prevention Study. Maturitas 2009;63:73–8.
26. Shah S, Carey I, Harris T, et al. Calcium supplementation, cardiovascular disease and mortality in older women. Pharmacoepidemiol Drug Saf 2010;19:59–64.
27. Hsu H, Culley N. Effects of dietary calcium on atherosclerosis, aortic calcification, and icterus in rabbits fed a supplemental cholesterol diet. Lipids Health Dis 2006; 5:16.
28. Bhakta M, Bruce C, Messika-Zeitoun D, et al. Oral calcium supplements do not affect the progression of aortic valve calcification or coronary artery calcification. J Am Board Fam Med 2009;22:610–6.
29. LaCroix A, Kotchen J, Anderson G, et al. Calcium plus vitamin D supplementation and mortality in postmenopausal women: the Women's Health Initiative calcium-vitamin D randomized controlled trial. J Gerontol 2009;64A:559–67.
30. Hsia L, Heiss G, Ren H. Calcium/vitamin D supplementation and cardiovascular events. Circulation 2007;115:845–52.
31. Yao S, Sucheston L, Millen A, et al. Pretreatment serum concentrations of 25-hydroxyvitamin D and breast cancer prognostic characteristics: a case-control and case-series study. PLoS One 2011;6:e17251.
32. Garland C, Gorham E, Mohr S, et al. Vitamin D and prevention of breast cancer: pooled analysis. J Steroid Biochem Mol Biol 2007;103:701–11.
33. Chen P, Hu P, Xie D, et al. Meta-analysis of vitamin D, calcium, and the prevention of breast cancer. Breast Cancer Res Treat 2010;121:469–77.
34. Gorman E, Garland C, Garland F, et al. Optimal vitamin D status for colorectal cancer prevention: a quantitative meta-analysis. Am J Prev Med 2007;32:210–6.
35. Touvier M, Chan D, Lau R, et al. Meta-analysis of vitamin D intake, 25-hydroxyvitamin D status, vitamin D receptor polymorphisms and colorectal cancer. Cancer Epidemiol Biomarkers Prev 2011;20(5):1003–16.
36. Raimondi S, Johansson H, Maisonneuve P, et al. Review and meta-analysis on vitamin D receptor polymorphisms and cancer risk. Carcinogenesis 2009;37: 1170–80.
37. Yin L, Grandi N, Raum E, et al. Meta-analysis: circulating vitamin D and ovarian cancer risk. Gynecol Oncol 2011;121(2):369–75.
38. Choo C, Mamedov A, Chung M, et al. Vitamin D insufficiency is common in patients with nonmetastatic prostate cancer. Nutr Res 2011;31:21–6.
39. Field S, Newton-Bishop J. Melanoma and vitamin D. Mol Oncol 2011;5(2): 197–214.
40. Bulathsinghala P, Syrigos K, Saif M. Role of vitamin D in the prevention of pancreatic cancer. J Nutr Metab 2011 [Epub ahead of print].
41. Zabiotska L, Gong Z, Wang F, et al. Vitamin D, calcium, and retinol intake, and pancreatic cancer in a population-based case-control study in the San Francisco Bay area. Cancer Causes Control 2011;22:91–100.

42. Broder A, Tobin J, Putterman C. Disease-specific definitions of vitamin D deficiency need to be established in autoimmune and non-autoimmune chronic diseases: a retrospective comparison of three chronic diseases. Arthritis Res Ther 2010;12:R191.
43. Guillot X, Semerano L, Saidenberg-Kermanac'h N, et al. Vitamin D and inflammation. Joint Bone Spine 2010;77:552–7.
44. Marques D, Dantas A, Fragoso T, et al. The importance of vitamin D levels in autoimmune disease. Rev Bras Rheumtol 2010;50:61–7.
45. Amital H, Szekanecz Z, Szucs G, et al. Serum concentrations of 25-OH vitamin D with systemic lupus erythematosis (SLE) are inversely related to disease activity: is it time to routinely supplement patients with SLE with vitamin D? Ann Rheum Dis 2010;69:1155–7.
46. Lee Y, Bae S, Choi S, et al. Associations between vitamin D receptor polymorphisms and susceptibility to rheumatoid arthritis and systemic lupus erythematosis: a meta-analysis. Mol Biol Rep 2011;38(6):3643–51.
47. Abbasi M, Rezaieyazdi Z, Afshari J, et al. Lack of association of vitamin D receptor gene BsmI polymorphisms in patient with systemic lupus erythematosis. Rheumatol Int 2010;30:1537–9.
48. Szodoray P, Tarr T, Bazso A, et al. The immunopathological role of vitamin D in patients with SLE: data from a single centre registry in Hungary. Scand J Rheumatol 2011;40:122–6.
49. Palomer X, Gonzalez-Clemente J, Blanco-Vaca F, et al. Role of vitamin D in the pathogenesis of type 2 diabetes mellitus. Diabetes Obes Metab 2008;10:185–97.
50. Takiishi T, Gysemans C, Boullion R, et al. Vitamin D and diabetes. Endocrinol Metab Clin North Am 2010;39:419–46.
51. Andizzone S, Cassinotti A, Bevilacqua M, et al. Vitamin D and inflammatory bowel disease. Vitam Horm 2011;86:367–77.
52. Brown A. The role of vitamin D in multiple sclerosis. Ann Pharmacother 2006;40:1158–61.
53. De Rezende Pena C, Grillo L, das Chagas Mederios M. Evaluation of 25-hydroxyvitamin D serum levels in patients with fibromyalgia. J Clin Rheumatol 2010;16:365–9.
54. Armstrong D, Meenegh GK, Bickle I, et al. Vitamin D deficiency is associated with anxiety and depression in fibromyalgia. Clin Rheumatol 2007;26:551–4.

Is There a Place for Bone Turnover Markers in the Assessment of Osteoporosis and its Treatment?

Jean-Pierre Devogelaer, MD[a],*, Yves Boutsen, MD[b],
Damien Gruson, CP[c], Daniel Manicourt, MD, PhD[a]

KEYWORDS

- Osteoporosis • Therapy • Biologic markers • Bone remodeling
- Bisphosphonates • Promotors of bone formation

Bone tissue is constantly remodeling in the adult skeleton. Bones must resist continuous different mechanical strains in daily life. The skeleton is influenced by various systemic hormonal stimuli. Moreover, local cytokines have a large role in bone turnover. It is generally considered that the skeleton is completely renewed every 10 years.

In normal circumstances in healthy adults, bone remodeling maintains bone mass as well as structural integrity and function. Moreover, it eventually adapts the skeleton to repetitive strains and injuries.[1] This mechanism results from the action of specialized cells: bone resorption by osteoclasts whose role consists of eliminating old bone that has become unfit for its mechanical and/or metabolic functions, and bone formation by osteoblasts to rebuild new bone. Buried cells (osteocytes) control the mechanostat, responding to skeletal strain by secreting sclerostin, which circulates through interconnected canaliculi and communicate with the bone surface. This process

The authors have nothing to disclose.

[a] Division of Rheumatology and Rheumatology Unit, Department of Medicine, UCL 5390, Université Catholique de Louvain in Brussels, Saint-Luc University Hospital, Avenue Hippocrate 10, B-1200 Brussels, Belgium

[b] Division of Rheumatology, Department of Medicine, UCL 5390, Université Catholique de Louvain in Brussels, Saint-Luc University Hospital, and University Hospital in Mont-Godinne, Avenue Dr Therasse 1, B-5530 Yvoir, Belgium

[c] Departments of Laboratory Medicine and Clinical Biochemistry, Université Catholique de Louvain in Brussels, Saint-Luc University Hospital, Avenue Hippocrate 10F, B-1200 Brussels, Belgium

* Corresponding author.
E-mail address: devogelaer@ruma.ucl.ac.be

Rheum Dis Clin N Am 37 (2011) 365–386
doi:10.1016/j.rdc.2011.07.002
0889-857X/11/$ – see front matter © 2011 Elsevier Inc. All rights reserved.

stimulates the remodeling cells mainly through the action of the RANKL-RANK-OPG cytokine system in the basic multicellular units (BMUs).[1] The normal rate of bone remodeling is still a matter of debate.[2] It is difficult to establish reference values that are validated worldwide for healthy premenopausal women. For example, serum carboxy-terminal crosslinking telopeptide of type I collagen (sCTX) was found to be significantly higher in France, relative to the United Kingdom, and procollagen type I N-terminal propeptide (PINP) was higher in France and Belgium compared with the United Kingdom and United States. This could be still different in other countries. About 2.5% of young, healthy, premenopausal women have levels of bone turnover markers (BTMs) less than the lower limit of any reference interval.[3] An International Osteoporosis Foundation (IOF) working group recently called for reference standards.

In normal postmenopausal women, the median remodeling period lasts about 8.2 months (range 3.4–54.0 months).[4] Both cellular actions are coupled in BMUs, which are 20 times more numerous in trabecular bone than in cortical bone (which represents 80% of the skeleton mass). These characteristics explain the more rapid changes in bone metabolism observed in trabecular bone than in cortical bone in circumstances with enhanced bone remodeling (eg, after menopause). Bone loss associated with postmenopause, aging, or pathologic conditions is caused by a negative balance between osteoblastic and osteoclastic activities, which can be amplified by the activation frequency of the remodeling units. Nowadays, the global level of bone remodeling can be estimated by several biologic BTMs. However, it is not possible to discriminate trabecular from cortical bone remodeling. In growing children, bone is modeling to adapt the shape of bones to their lengthening, and is also remodeling (as for adults). It is also not possible to discriminate between modeling and remodeling with BTMs in children.

It has recently been suggested that bone fragility can at least partly be assessable independently of bone mineral density (BMD) by measuring bone remodeling activity with some BTMs.[5]

Osteoporosis (OP) is a systemic skeletal condition characterized by low bone mass and microarchitectural deterioration of bone tissue, with a consequent increase in bone fragility and susceptibility to fracture.[6] It is nowadays easy to measure BMD, and this led a World Health Organization (WHO) study group to define intervention definitions for OP based on the BMD assessment by dual-energy X ray absorptiometry (DXA).[7,8] Contrary to BMD measurement, the microarchitecture assessment until recently exclusively needed the analysis of transilial bone biopsies by histomorphometry. Microcomputed tomography (μCT) and high-resolution magnetic resonance imaging (hrMRI), able to assess microarchitecture in vivo and atraumatically, are in development. They are not yet used clinically on a large scale.

FRAX is a new tool adopted by WHO and based on simple clinical risk factors such as age, weight, height, body mass index (BMI), personal or parental fracture history, secondary causes of OP, glucocorticoid (GC) use, smoking habits, and alcohol (ab) use. FRAX provides an estimation of the 10-year probability percentage of OP fractures (hip and major OP fractures).[9] With the use of FRAX, either alone or in conjunction with DXA measurements, the indication for OP therapy should be refined.

BMD is an excellent predictor of the fracture risk based on large prospective studies.[10] BMD measurements necessitate at least 1 to 2 years for quantifiable changes caused by therapeutic agents. However, it is not available everywhere. FRAX has the advantages of being clinically easily assessable and being adaptable to country-specific fracture risks. It can also be upgraded.[11,12] FRAX is not modified by any therapy, however. Falls, particularly those that threaten to fracture if they are frequent, are not included in the FRAX tool assessment and need a personalized clinical judgment. Furthermore, a large study on risedronate (RIS) treatment did not show reduction of the risk of hip fracture in elderly women whose selection had only been based on nonskeletal (clinical) risk factors. The decrease in fracture risk was exclusively observed in patients with low BMD in this study.[13] In the Nordic Research on Ageing (NORA) study, 82% of postmenopausal women with fractures had T-scores higher than − 2.5, but this was only based on appendicular bone densitometry.[14] Thus, even if a therapeutic indication is based on FRAX and BMD measurements, several patients at risk may still not be considered for therapy.

Biochemical indices of bone remodeling provide dynamic information about bone status, regarding the bone turnover rate. They are central to the mechanisms involved both directly and indirectly in the mechanical resistance of the skeleton (**Fig. 1**). Furthermore, they can change rapidly, in a few days to weeks following the action of potent antiosteoporotic therapies. They have been of utmost value in the development of new therapies for OP and have been largely used in trials involving thousands of patients, which have rendered them more familiar to the clinicians. However, the extrapolation of the trial data to the management of an individual patient is still questionable. Taking everything into account, the main questions are whether there is a place for BTMs in OP assessment, and whether BTMs are a further means to identify patients at risk of fracture.

CHARACTERISTICS OF BTMs

The general characteristics of BTMs are summarized in **Box 1**. The high level of BTMs with aging is not only explained by the progressive age-related decline in the glomerular filtration rate inducing an increase in parathyroid hormone (PTH) levels. It could be partly explained, at least for urinary markers, by sarcopenia, which is accompanied by a decrease in the urinary excretion of creatinine, a denominator that, as an artifact, increases the urine BTM levels, which are corrected by creatinine.[15] Most BTMs have a circadian rhythm, being high during the night and

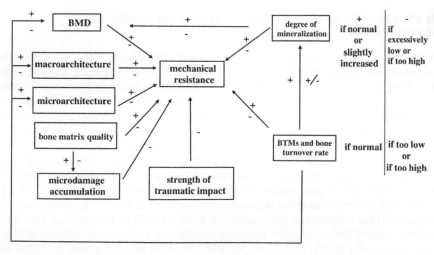

BMD = bone mineral density, BTMs (bone turnover markers)

Fig. 1. Theoretic determinants of bone fragility.

Box 1
General characteristics of BTMs

- Increase after menopause in most women
- Possible increase in late premenopause and in perimenopause (when irregular menses and FSH are increased)
- No age-related decline
- Circadian rhythm (high during the night and in the morning, low in the afternoon)
- Seasonal variation as for BMD, partly caused by low winter levels of 25OHD$_3$, with secondary hyperparathyroidism
- Long-term increase after fracture, up to 1 year, particularly of the hip[23]

Data from Refs.[15–23]

---

in the morning and low in the afternoon. There is a seasonal variation in BMD,[16] as well as in the parameters of bone remodeling, partly caused by low winter levels of 25OHD$_3$, inducing some degree of secondary hyperparathyroidism. The seasonal changes are possibly preventable by high dietary calcium and vitamin D or by supplementation.[17–20] Long-term potassium citrate supplementation is not capable of reducing bone turnover or of provoking any increase in BMD values in healthy postmenopausal women.[21] Therefore, alkali supplementation does not constitute an explanation for the apparent good effect of fruit and vegetable on bone.[22] BTMs can remain increased for up to 1 year after a fracture, particularly of the hip.[23] The BTMs clinically available to measure bone formation and bone resorption are summarized in **Tables 1** and **2**. There is currently no means to recommend the use of a particular BTM in daily practice. Recently, an IOF working group suggested the use of 2 markers in clinical trials, sCTX, a marker of bone resorption, and PINP, a marker of bone formation.

CAN BTMs BE USED AS ALTERNATIVE MARKERS IN THE DIAGNOSIS OF OSTEOPOROSIS?

Before menopause and in women within 20 years of menopause, less than 10% of the variability of both total body bone mineral content (BMC) and lumbar, hip, and distal radius BMD could be accounted for by the markers of bone remodeling.[15] Later, BTMs could explain up to 52% of the BMD variance in a large group of women with increasing time after menopause.[15] In a smaller group of postmenopausal women, Marcus and colleagues[24] observed that both age and BMI at baseline taken together accounted for 16% and 25% of the variance of baseline BMD of the spine and of the hip, respectively. The addition of baseline urinary amino-terminal crosslinking telopeptide of type I collagen (uNTX), or urinary carboxy-terminal crosslinking telopeptide of type I collagen (uCTX) and serum bone specific alkaline phosphatase (sBSAP), to age and BMI only increased the regression values to 22% and 28%, respectively. In this study, BTMs offered little information for estimating BMD in individual women.[24] In elderly, healthy French women, negative correlations were found between sBSAP, serum osteocalcin (sOC), uCTX and hip BMD.[25] However, there was no threshold value fit for use to diagnose OP. Therefore, BTMs cannot currently constitute alternatives for BMD in the diagnosis of OP in individual patients.

ARE BTMs AN INDEPENDENT RISK FACTOR FOR FRACTURE RISK ASSESSMENT?

It is well accepted that a decrease in BMD by 1 T score entails approximately a twofold increase in the relative risk of spinal, hip, and forearm fracture.[10] Resorption BTMs could predict fractures of the spine and of the hip independently from BMD.[26–28] An association has also been reported between markers of bone formation and the risk of fracture.[27,29,30] Low levels of undercarboxylated osteocalcin, compatible with a low vitamin K level, were also found to be accompanied by an increased risk of hip fracture.[31,32] BMD and BTMs could constitute independent fracture risk factors. In the OFELY study, the 5-year relative fracture risks associated with an isolated low BMD or with an isolated high CTX were less increased than both low BMD and high CTX combined (respectively 39%, 25%, and 55%), suggesting that they did not select the same patients, notwithstanding some overlapping.[27] In a recent study of 1040 75-year-old women, baseline levels of BTMs, high serum tartrate-resistant acid phosphatase (sTRACP) 5B and sCTX were associated with an increased risk of any kind of fracture (hazard ratio [HR] and 95% confidence interval [CI] of 1.16 and 1.04, 1.29; 1.13 and 1.01, 1.27, respectively per increase of 1 standard deviation [SD] in these parameters). HRs for clinical vertebral fracture were also increased (1.22, 95% CI 1.01, 1.48; and 1.32, 95% CI 1.05, 1.67, respectively), but not for hip fractures. The predictive value of BTMs was maintained longer for vertebral fractures (at least for 5 years).[28]

However, in an individual patient suffering from OP, BTMs cannot yet be used for the indication of therapy, contrary to low BMD values with or without the use of the FRAX tool. It is not known whether the addition of BTMs to the calculation of the simple and inexpensive FRAX tool could significantly improve the predictive value of the latter.

Osteopenia, defined by a BMD T score between less than −1 and greater than −2.5, a theoretic condition between normals and osteoporosis, has not been recognized as an indication for therapy in most countries, even if most of fractures occur in patients with a T score greater than −2.5.[14] In the OFELY study, a 10-year probability of fracture of 26% could be measured in patients with osteopenia only when 1 risk factor among age, high BSAP and a prior fracture was also present, compared with only 6% in women with a osteopenic BMD value as the sole risk factor.[29] At that time, the FRAX tool was not yet available, and the magnitude of increase in risk that could have been added to the clinical risk factors by BTMs is not known. In the EPIDOS study, another study from the Lyon group, morning serum CTX was not accompanied by an increased risk of hip fractures. When restricted to samples taken between 1 and 2 PM, a time schedule for sampling that is usually not recommended, the relative hazard for hip fracture amounted to 1.86 for values of CTX 2 SDs more than the premenopausal mean value.[33] These relative inconsistencies led the WHO Task Force on FRAX to not implement BTMs as a risk factor owing to the absence of global data and variability of the techniques (S. Silverman, personal communication, 2011).

Future prospective studies are necessary to determine whether, in addition to BMD measurements and the use of the FRAX tool, BTMs could find significant numbers of patients with osteopenia, justifying pharmacologic therapy.

Moreover, in men aged 50 to 85 years followed for an average of 7.5 years, the correlations between BTMs and the rate of BMD loss seemed to be weak, the variability of BTMs explaining less than 2% of the bone loss variability. Furthermore, there was no prediction of incident fractures by BTM levels.[34] However, in a recent study, it was shown that, before the age of 70 years, microarchitecture of bone assessed by high-resolution peripheral quantitative computed tomography at distal radius and tibia only weakly depended on the current rate bone turnover, contrary to what was observed in older men.[35]

Table 1
Biomarkers related to bone resorption: available assays, sampling precautions, preanalytical factors, and analytical and biologic variability

Biomarker	Available Assay Format	Sampling	Preanalytical Variability	Analytical Variability	Biologic Variability
CTX	ECLIA ELISA	Serum Urine	Morning collection after overnight fast Urine: second morning void	Intralaboratory within-run CV about 10% Intralaboratory between-run CV about 12% Interlaboratory CV ND	Circadian rhythm Food intake Age Gender Fractures Pregnancy Kidney function If urinary measurement, must be corrected with urinary creatinine levels Intraindividual variability about 10%
iCTP or CTX-MMP	ELISA	Serum	Morning collection after overnight fast	Intralaboratory within-run CV about 10% Intralaboratory between-run CV about 10% Interlaboratory CV 25%	Circadian rhythm Food intake Age Gender Fractures Pregnancy Kidney function Intraindividual variability ND
NTX	ELISA ECi	Serum Urine	Morning collection Urine: second morning void	Intralaboratory within-run CV about 10% Intralaboratory between-run CV about 10% Interlaboratory CV 40% (urine)	Circadian rhythm Food intake Age Gender Fractures Pregnancy If urinary measurement, must be corrected with urinary creatinine levels Intraindividual variability about 10%

DPD	ELISA RIA	Urine	Morning collection Avoid exposure to ultraviolet light Second morning void	Intralaboratory within-run CV about 15% Intralaboratory between-run CV about 15% Interlaboratory CV 25%	Circadian rhythm Age Gender Fractures Pregnancy Measurement must be corrected with urinary creatinine levels Intraindividual variability about 20%
PYD	ELISA RIA	Urine	Morning collection Avoid exposure to ultraviolet light Second morning void	Intralaboratory within-run CV about 15% Intralaboratory between-run CV about 15% Interlaboratory CV 25%	Circadian rhythm Age Gender Fractures Pregnancy Liver function Active arthritis Measurement must be corrected with urinary creatinine levels Intraindividual variability about 20%
TRACP	ELISA	Serum	Avoid hemolysis	Intralaboratory within-run CV about 10% Intralaboratory between-run CV about 10% Interlaboratory CV ND	Circadian rhythm Age Gender Fractures Intraindividual variability about 25%
HYP	HPLC method	Urine	Second morning void Keep samples refrigerated or frozen until analysis	Intralaboratory within-run CV about 15% Intralaboratory between-run CV about 15% Interlaboratory CV ND	Nonspecific for bone Affected by food intake Measurement must be corrected with urinary creatinine levels Intraindividual variability ND

Abbreviations: CV, coefficient of variation; ICTP or CTX-MMP, carboxy-terminal crosslinking telopeptide of type I collagen generated by matrixmetalloproteinases; CTX, carboxy-terminal crosslinking telopeptide of type I collagen; DPD, deoxypyridinoline; ECLIA, electrochemiluminescent immunoassay; ELISA, enzyme-linked immunosorbent assay; ECi, enhanced chemiluminescent assay; HYP, hydroxyproline; HPLC, high performance liquid chromatography; ND, not documented; NTX, amino-terminal crosslinking telopeptide of type I collagen; PYD, pyridinoline; RIA, radioimmunoassay; TRACP, tartrate-resistant acid phosphatase.

Table 2
Biomarkers related to bone formation: available assays, sampling precautions, preanalytical, analytical and biologic variability

Biomarker	Available Assays	Sampling	Preanalytical Variability	Analytical Variability	Biologic Variability
PINP	ECLIA ELISA RIA	Serum	Stable biomarker No specific need of fasting	Intralaboratory within-run CV about 10% Intralaboratory between-run CV about 10% Interlaboratory CV ND	Circadian rhythm (low) Age Gender Fractures Pregnancy Intraindividual variability about 12%
PICP	ELISA RIA	Serum	Poorly documented	Intralaboratory within-run CV about 10% Intralaboratory between-run CV about 10% Interlaboratory CV ND	Circadian rhythm (low) Age Gender Fractures Pregnancy Intraindividual variability ND
BSAP	CLIA ELISA	Serum	Keep samples refrigerated or frozen until analysis Avoid hemolysis	Intralaboratory within-run CV about 10% Intralaboratory between-run CV about 10% Interlaboratory CV 30%	Circadian rhythm (low) Age Gender Fractures Pregnancy Intraindividual variability about 8%
OC	CLIA ELISA ECLIA	Serum Urine	Keep samples frozen until analysis to avoid degradation Avoid hemolysis Urine, second morning void	Intralaboratory within-run CV about 10% Intralaboratory between-run CV about 15% Interlaboratory CV 40%	Circadian rhythm Kidney function Age Gender Fractures Pregnancy If urinary measurement, must be corrected with urinary creatinine levels Intraindividual variability about 20%

Abbreviations: BSAP, bone-specific alkaline phosphatase; CLIA, chemiluminescent immunoassay; CV, coefficient of variation; ECLIA, electrochemiluminescent immunoassay; ELISA, enzyme-linked immunosorbent assay; ND, not documented; OC, osteocalcin; PICP, procollagen type I carboxy-terminal propeptide; PINP, procollagen type I amino-terminal propeptide; RIA, radioimmunoassay.

Type 1 diabetes is accompanied by a reduced BMD in men, osteopenia and osteoporosis in our experience being observed in 33% and 7% of patients, respectively.[36] A negative significant correlation was found between lumbar BMD and sCTX ($r = -0.343$). However, a positive correlation between lumbar BMD and age was also observed ($r = 0.365$), not linked to degenerative changes. A similar trend was observed at the hip. Osteoprotegerin was significantly increased in diabetic patients compared with age-matched controls, and positively correlated with age ($r = 0.507$), contrary to sCTX ($r = -0.39$). These results suggest an inhibition of osteoclast activation and a reduced bone resorption with age in men suffering from type 1 diabetes.[36]

DO BTMs PREDICT POSTMENOPAUSAL BONE LOSS?

In normal young adults, there is an equilibrium between the resorption of old bone by osteoclasts and the new bone formation by the osteoblasts.

After menopause, because of the decrease in estrogen secretion, there is an acceleration of turnover leading to an increase of both bone formation and bone resorption with an enhanced activation frequency of BMUs. However, bone formation cannot compete with the dramatic increase in the number of resorption lacunae, and the increase in bone formation is unable to replace all the resorbed bone when turnover accelerates. The resorption lacunae become more and more numerous and deeper, and perforations of the trabeculae take place. A bone loss at the BMU levels results, macroscopically measurable by bone densitometry. Perforations of the trabeculae lead to a loss of connectivity that further reduces the strength of bone to a larger order of magnitude than is predicted by the decrease in BMD alone. BTM levels increase rapidly. An increase of up to +79% to +97% in the parameters of bone resorption (NTX and CTX) and of up to 37%–52% of bone formation (serum OC and BSAP) has been observed, with long-term persistence of high remodeling until up to 40 years after menopause.[15] However, baseline levels of BTMs were only weakly correlated with the 5-year whole-body BMD loss.[37] Except for sBSAP, the correlation was found to be a little better between BTMs and BMD measured at the legs, with no clear superiority of one specific marker or group of markers in a Scandinavian study.[38] Several longitudinal studies confirm that, in groups of patients with persistently high bone turnover, there is a more rapid bone loss than in groups with normal or low bone turnover.[37–42] Observed percentages of bone loss according to the level of bone turnover are shown in **Table 3**. The correlations were better between BTMs and appendicular bone loss, particularly with serial assessments of BTMs showing a constant high

Table 3
Observed percentage of BMD loss in postmenopausal women according to the level of turnover

	Total Body BMD Loss (%)	Hip BMD Loss (%)
Constantly high bone turnover	−2.6	−8.3
Intermediate turnover	−1.6	−6.0
Low bone turnover	−0.2	−5.1

Data from Ivaska KK, Lenora J, Gerdhem P, et al. Serial assessment of serum bone metabolism markers identifies women with the highest rate of bone loss and osteoporosis risk. J Clin Endocrinol Metab 2008;93:2622–32.

turnover. Degenerative changes in the spine can, as an artifact, increase lumbar BMD measurements.[37] Even if there exist significant correlations between BMD loss and BTMs in groups of postmenopausal women, stronger close to menopause and early postmenopause, the scatter of individual values of BMD loss is large for an equivalent BTM level, so that it is not reasonable to use BTMs as predictors for BMD and BMD loss in an individual woman.[43] Moreover, if the repetition of BTM measurements significantly improves their predictive value, their cost/benefit will be questioned if they just serve to predict bone loss.

DO BTMs HELP IN THE CHOICE OF A SPECIFIC THERAPY?

In theory, a better response to antiresorptive agents would be expected in patients with a high rate compared with patients having a low rate of bone turnover, and an inverse situation for the therapeutic response to the promoters of bone formation. However, this is not always observed in therapeutic trials.

Antiresorptive Agents

Higher pretreatment levels of bone turnover conferred a higher response in BMD while on antiresorptive agents, notably with oral alendronate (ALN), intravenous (IV) pamidronate (PAM), and estrogen replacement therapy (ERT).[44,45] However, any baseline level of urine deoxypyridinoline (uDPD) conferred a similar spine antifracture efficacy in the treated group in an analysis of pooled RIS trials.[46] This observation was the exception rather than the rule. In the Fracture Intervention Trial (FIT) , a post hoc analysis showed that a high pretreatment level of PINP conferred a better nonspine fracture efficacy (but not spine) to ALN therapy.[45] Each SD reduction in the 1-year percent change in BSAP was associated with a 26% (95% CI 13–37) decrease in spine fracture, 11% (0–22) in nonspine fracture, and 39% (20–54) in hip fracture. The respective numbers were 33% (10–34), 10% (3–20), 22% (+19 to −49), and 17% (5–27), 6% (+6 to −16), and 11% (+31 to −39), respectively for PINP and sCTX. Comparative values for an increase in BMD of 2.6% at total hip after 1 year were 36% (11–39) for spine fracture, 3% (+17 to −10) for nonspine fracture, and 26% (+17 to −53) for hip fracture.[47]

However, as mentioned earlier, more than half of fractures occur in postmenopausal women with a BMD T score higher than − 2.5 (ie, suffering from osteopenia).[14] It is possible that the use of BTMs could detect patients more susceptible to a cost-effective antifracture efficacy to antiresorptive agents, as suggested in a Markov model.[48] Future prospective clinical studies will have to confirm the data of this theoretic model.

Promotors of Bone Formation

In the Fracture Prevention Trial, a significant positive correlation was observed in postmenopausal women treated with subcutaneous (s/c) teriparatide-20 (TPTD) between the baseline bone turnover status (sBSAP; $r = 0.28$), sPICP (procollagen type I C-terminal propeptide; $r = 0.36$), sPINP ($r = 0.41$), free uDPD ($r = 0.23$), and uNTX ($r = 0.40$) and the BMD response at the lumbar spine after 18 months. The respective correlations with the hip BMD changes after 12 months were much worse.[49]

In a study on GC-OP, baseline serum OC concentrations were less than the lower limit of the normal reference range in about one-third of patients, underlying the reduced osteoblast function.[50] During TPTD therapy, they were still 13%, 12%, 10%, and 23%, with values of OC less than the reference range after 1, 6, 18, and 36 months, respectively.[50] Increases in lumbar spine and femoral neck BMD induced by TPTD were not significantly correlated with baseline marker concentrations (sβCTX, PINP, PICP, BSAP). In contrast, in the ALN group, the increase in femoral neck BMD at 18 months was positively correlated with the baseline concentrations of all markers.[50] This could possibly be because, contrary to ALN, the TPTD response was partially blunted in patients receiving high doses of GC.[51,52] However, there was a significant correlation between the changes in PINP at 1 and 6 months and the changes in both the femoral neck (r = 0.34 and 0.30) and lumbar spine BMD (r = 0.33 and 0.23), respectively. In the ALN group, there was a significant correlation between the decrease in sCTX after 1 month and the increase in lumbar BMD after 18 months (r = −0.32), and between the decrease in PINP and βCTX after 1 and 6 months and the increase in femoral neck BMD at 18 months.

According to the available data, even if the initial levels of the parameters of bone remodeling are correlated with the BMD response (inversely correlated for the use of bisphosphonates [BPs], and directly for TPTD), there are not sufficient data for the antifracture efficacy. Only post hoc analysis for ALN, RIS, and ibandronate (IBA) suggested a correlation between a decrease of greater than 30% in BTMs and spine and nonspine fracture prevention.[45,47,53–55] Case by case, the clinician in charge of the patient could decide to measure BTMs if the patient is reluctant to maintain therapy in spite of repetitive discussions, but an unconsidered use of BTMs in every case to prove a therapeutic response is not currently recommended.

ROLE OF BTMs IN THE PREDICTION OF THERAPEUTIC RESPONSE
Changes in BMD

In a meta-analysis of 12 trials of therapy with antiresorptive agents, compared with the data from FIT, it was estimated that the increase in BMD produced by antiresorptive agents accounted, at most, for a decrease in fracture risk of about 20%, whereas most of the trials showed a reduction of fracture risk of the order of 45% or more.[56] This emphasizes a potential role for BTMs. The inhibition of bone remodeling is itself another important mechanism explaining the rapid improvement of the fracture rate (within a few months), therefore not simply attributable to the much slower increase in BMD. Because there is a coupling between resorption and formation in bone remodeling, a therapy with antiresorptive agents will at term decrease both parameters of bone resorption and bone formation (**Fig. 2**). However, there is some delay between the rapid and abrupt reduction in parameters of resorption, and the later and less marked decrease of bone formation parameters. This process allows for the steep increase in BMD during the first months. The increase in BMD is attributable to the refilling of the resorption lacunae by new bone that is rapidly mineralized. As the remodeling slows down, more time is left for the secondary mineralization, which becomes more complete. The BMD continues to increase, but at a slower pace, or can even level off according to the bone compartments (trabecular or cortical) (**Fig. 3**).[57] Examples of the changes observed in bone markers following therapy with antiosteoporotic drugs are shown in **Table 4**.

In contrast with antiresorptive agents, TPTD induced an increase in parameters of bone resorption and of bone formation, the latter being more marked (see **Fig. 2**).

The effect of TPTD is rapid (within a few days). PINP has been shown to be already increasing rapidly 2 days after the start of therapy with TPTD, and it continued to increase until the end of 28 days' treatment in a short study in osteopenic postmenopausal women.[58] The increase in PICP and OC was a little less marked.

Such an early response of the markers of bone formation to TPTD is predictive of the BMD response in postmenopausal women with OP. The increases observed in PICP

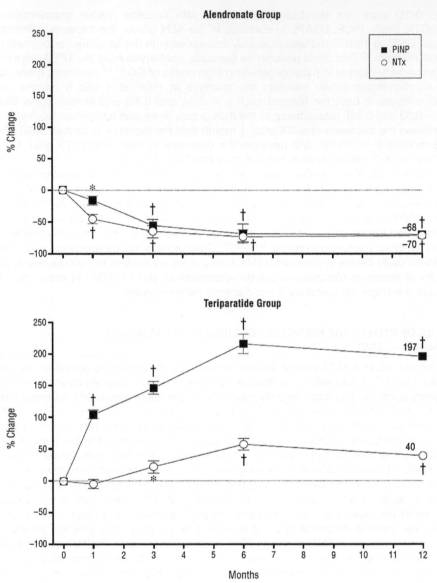

Fig. 2. Percentage change (mean ± standard error [SE]) from baseline in serum PINP and urinary N-telopeptide corrected for creatinine (NTx) in the alendronate and teriparatide treatment groups. Asterisk indicates P<.05; dagger, P<.001. (*From* McClung MR, San Martin J, Miller PD, et al. Opposite bone remodeling effects of teriparatide and alendronate in increasing bone mass. Arch Intern Med 2005;165:1764. Copyright © 2005 American Medical Association. All rights reserved; with permission.)

at 1 month and in PINP after 3 months significantly correlated with lumbar spine BMD increases after 18 months (r = 0.65 and 0.61, respectively).[49] Sixty-eight percent of patients were considered responders (≥3% BMD increase at L-BMD after 18 months), 8% definite nonresponders (BMD decrease of >3%), and 24% indeterminate

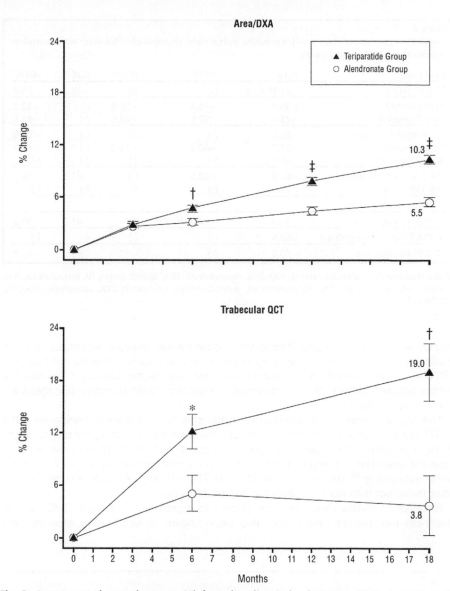

Fig. 3. Percentage change (mean ± SE) from baseline in lumbar spine BMD. Asterisk indicates *P*<.05; dagger, *P*<.01; and double dagger, *P*<.001 (alendronate vs teriparatide for all). Difference between the action of a promoter of bone formation (*upper curves*) and an antiresorptive agent (*lower curves*). Areal DXA (posteroanterior) measures the integral BMD (both cortical and trabecular bone together), whereas QCT can measure separately cortical and trabecular bone BMD. The gain in trabecular BMD observed with teriparatide (TPTD) amounted to more than 2-times that observed with alendronate (ALN) after 6 months. Later on, between 6 and 18 months, ALN no longer produced any increase in trabecular lumbar BMD, whereas TPTD therapy continued to induce trabecular lumbar BMD gain, up to 5-times greater compared with ALN. (*From* McClung MR, San Martin J, Miller PD, et al. Opposite bone remodeling effects of teriparatide and alendronate in increasing bone mass. Arch Intern Med 2005;165:1765. Copyright © 2005 American Medical Association. All rights reserved; with permission.)

Table 4
Order of magnitude of the mean (or median) percentage changes of BTMs after antiresorptive agents therapy for 1 to 2 years

Oral Drug	sCTX	uNTX	sPINP	sOC	sBSAP
RAL 60 mg/d	−27.8(uCTX)	(-)	(-)	−28.3	−29.0
ALN 10 mg/d	−59.2	−73.4	−50.9	(-)	−43.1
ALN 70 mg/wk	−73.8	−52.8	−63.9	(-)	−40.6
RIS 5 mg/d (median)	−55.0	(-)	(-)	(-)	−35.0
RIS 35 mg/wk	−54.7	−40.3	−48.0	(-)	−28.1
RIS 150 mg/mo	−50.0	(-)	(-)	(-)	(-)
IBA 2.5 mg/d (median)	−62.6	−60.5	(-)	−51.5	−38.1
IBA 150 mg/mo	−75.8	(-)	(-)	(-)	(-)
Parenteral drug					
IV-ZOL 5 mg/y	−59.0	−58.0(sNTX)	(-)	−45.0	−30.0
IV-IBA 3 mg/3 mo (median)	−58.6	(-)	(-)	(-)	(-)
s/c DSB 60 mg/6 mo	−80.0	(-)	−70.0	(-)	−40.0

Abbreviations: ALN, alendronate; d, day; DSB, denosumab; IBA, ibandronate; IV, intravenous; mo, months; RAL, raloxifene; RIS, risedronate; s/c, subcutaneous; wk, week; ZOL, zoledronic acid; (-), not found.

responders ($\geq$−3% but <3%).[49] However, the biomarker changes in nonresponders in BMD were approximately as large as in the good responders, showing not only that TPTD was administered but also that it was active on bone metabolism.[59] The reasons for the apparent difference in the therapeutic response could be many, and these are summarized in **Box 2**.[59,60]

The poor association between the biomarker changes and the BMD response in the TPTD therapy precludes their use in clinical medicine for predicting the responses to therapy. However, the positive correlation of spine and hip BMD response with the baseline rate of remodeling suggests that TPTD is more active in patients with active bone remodeling.[59] The blunting effect on TPTD or PTH (1–84) action during and/or after treatment with ALN suggests the same conclusion.[61,62]

Strontium ranelate (SR) has been shown to significantly increase BMD and to decrease the fracture rate. It has also been shown to significantly stimulate the

Box 2
Theoretic reasons for a difference between the BMD response to teriparatide and BTM changes

- There was imprecision in the BMD measurement
- The BMD change was close to 0; without treatment, a BMD loss would have been observed
- TPTD could have induced an increase in the total bone area, thus reducing the BMD increase (BMD by DXA is BMC/area)

Data from Heaney RP, Watson P. Variability in the measured response of bone to teriparatide. Osteoporos Int 2010. [Epub ahead of print]; and Zanchetta JR, Bogado CE, Ferretti JL, et al. Effects of teriparatide [recombinant human parathyroid hormone (1–34)] on cortical bone in postmenopausal women with osteoporosis. J Bone Miner Res 2003;18:539–43.

parameters of bone formation (sBSAP+8.1%) after 3 months and to decrease the parameters of bone resorption (sCTX−12.5%), leading to some uncoupling in bone remodeling (**Fig. 4**).[63] These changes were maintained for 3 years. In a post hoc study of 2373 postmenopausal women, the short-term (3 months) changes in PICP and sBSAP, but not in sCTX or sNTX, were weakly but significantly associated with 3-year changes in lumbar spine BMD, at femoral neck and at total hip BMD, in an univariate analysis. Changes in both sBSAP and in sPICP were associated with changes in femoral neck BMD, and in total hip BMD only for PICP.[64] Less than 10% of the BMD changes were explained by the changes in biochemical markers. Moreover, the short-term changes in BTMs were not related to fractures. The changes in the markers after 3 months of treatment with SR therefore cannot be used in the individual patient to assess its efficacy on BMD changes.[64]

Comparing the effects of daily s/c injections of 100 μg PTH (1–84) and oral SR (2 g), there was, after 24 weeks, a dramatic increase in PINP with large scatters (+112.9 ± 101.2%) and BSAP (+18.8 ± 29.7%) from week 4 onwards in the PTH group, versus no significant change in the SR group, suggesting differing modes of anabolic action

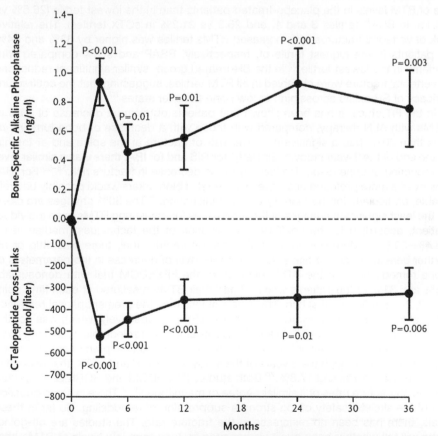

Fig. 4. SR-induced changes in serum biochemical markers of bone metabolism. Uncoupling phenomenon: increase in bone-specific alkaline phosphatase and decrease in C-telopeptide cross-links. (*From* Meunier PJ, Roux C, Seeman E, et al. The effects of strontium ranelate on the risk of vertebral fracture in women with postmenopausal osteoporosis. N Engl J Med 2004;350:465; with permission.)

of both drugs on bone remodeling.[65] It therefore seems that it is not advisable to use the biomarkers in individuals to predict the BMD response to TPTD and/or to SR.

Efficacy in Fracture Prevention

Raloxifene (RAL), a selective estrogen receptor modulator (SERM) produced a marginal increase after 3 years in lumbar spine BMD (+2.7%) and in femoral neck BMD (+2.4%) at the recommended dose of 60 mg/d. These modest changes in BMD were not related to vertebral fracture risk.[66] In the MORE study, it was shown that decreases of 9.3 µg/L in sOC and of 5.91 µg/L in sBSAP after 1 year of therapy were accompanied by an odds ratio (OR) for a new vertebral fracture during 3 years of 0.69 and 0.75, respectively. The predictive value of bone turnover changes was of similar magnitude compared with the predictive value of baseline BMD during raloxifene treatment.[66]

A progressive reduction in lumbar spine and femoral neck BMD was observed with increasing tertiles of baseline levels of BSAP and sCTX in more than 4891 postmenopausal women with OP in another post hoc analysis in the placebo group of study with SR therapy.[67] The incident vertebral fractures were more numerous in the highest tertile of BTM levels in the placebo-treated patients than in the lowest tertile (26.5% vs 21.1% in BSAP tertiles 3 and 1, and 26.3 vs 21.2% in sCTX tertiles). The relative risk of vertebral fractures with increased BTMs tertiles was higher by 32% and 24% in patients in the highest tertile of, respectively, BSAP and sCTX compared with patients in the lowest tertile.[67] In the SR-treated group, similar significant reductions in vertebral fracture were observed in all BTM tertiles, suggesting that the antifracture efficacy of SR exists across high or low bone turnover states.[67]

In the FIT study, it has been shown that patients obtaining a decrease of 30% in BTMs with ALN therapy, compared with those with a decrease of bone turnover of less than 30%, had a significantly lower risk of fracture at the spine and at the hip at the end of the 3-year study.[47] Similarly, for RIS and for IBA, there was a similar level of reduction of bone resorption leading to the decrease in fracture risk.[53-55] For IBA, however, a more profound decrease in the level of biomarkers would possibly be preferable, particularly for the monthly oral administration.[68] The 30% changes are close to the least significant changes of the techniques for measuring BTMs in an individual patient, according to the coefficient of variation of the techniques (median value 13.4%–20.6%). Moreover, in the RIS vertebral fracture trial, there was little or no further benefit in fracture risk at less than this level of decrease in the parameters of bone remodeling.[54] In the BTM substudy of the FREEDOM trial with denosumab, 46% and 31% of the patients who had had their BTMs measured at each time point (6, 12, 24, and 36 months) had BTM levels of less than the premenopausal reference interval from 6 months onward for sCTX and sPINP, respectively, which was not the case for TRACP5b or BSAP.[69] In the HORIZON study with zoledronic acid (5 mg IV/y), approximately 19% of patients had PINP levels of less than the premenopausal reference interval all through the 3 years of the study. For BSAP and sCTX, the respective numbers were 1.7% and 17.8%.[70] Both studies (FREEDOM and HORIZON) reported results on fracture rates of a similar degree of magnitude.[71,72] There is some question about the skeletal safety of too strong a suppression of remodeling. So far in these trials, there has been no reincrease in the fracture rate. The studies are on-going. Time will tell whether bone quality is impaired by long-term low levels of BTMs after antiresorptive therapies. About 2.5% of premenopausal women have BTMs levels of less than the premenopausal reference interval.[3] They evidently do not have other risk factors, such as falls and low BMD, compared with postmenopausal women. It is therefore difficult to individualize the threshold of BTM decrease to obtain an optimal long-term effect on the skeleton.[73] Further studies are necessary to determine the more efficient and safer threshold. Moreover, these studies should help to determine the most appropriate BTM(s), if any, to use in clinical practice.

PERSISTENCE ON THERAPY, AND PREVENTION OF COMPLICATIONS

As for most chronic diseases, persistence on therapy in OP is poor. It has been observed that about 50% of patients discontinue their treatment within 1 year.[74] In this recent study, only 35%, 25%, and 14% were still on oral therapy after 2, 3, and 4 years, respectively. The 3-year fracture incidence was inversely correlated with the length of adherence to therapy. This finding underlines the hazards of a poor compliance. It is theoretically possible that BTMs could be of some help in improving therapeutic adherence. However, in a study, the supplying of complementary information stressing the usefulness of adherence for the efficacy of therapy by nursing staff was at least equivalent to the use of BTMs for the therapeutic maintenance (+57%), compared with no information at all.[75] Therefore, in an individual case, regular information regarding the necessity of a strict adherence to therapy is crucial.

The ideal duration of BP therapy in a patient suffering from OP is difficult to determine. There are 2 studies reporting the use of ALN for up to 10 years.[57,76] Owing to the long retention time of BPs in the skeleton, it could be tempting to stop therapy after 3 or 5 years (the mean durations of the pivotal double-blind studies having shown a significant decrease in the fracture risk vs placebo). It has been suggested that weaning from treatment could be safe for 1 year, and maybe for longer, as far as the risk for hip fracture was concerned, provided the adherence to therapy before weaning was of good quality.[77] However, all BPs do not have a similar skeletal retention time, and, if the compliance to the drug was not the most appropriate, the risk of fracture could reincrease more rapidly after cessation of the drug. If they remain sufficiently abated, BTMs could help to estimate whether some protection by low bone turnover persists. For example, it has been shown with an IV injection of zoledronic acid that its antiresorptive action could persist for up to 2 years.[78] So far, no study has definitely shown the safety of this kind of BTM use or determined the appropriate BTMs level.

There have been suggestions that complications such as atypical subtrochanteric fractures and osteonecrosis of the jaw (ONJ) could be caused by too strong an inhibition of bone turnover by BPs, to the extent that normal bone repair was altered.[79,80] However, the ability of BTMs, notably of CTX, to be a valuable predictor of ONJ has not been validated in large prospective clinical trials. Furthermore, a decrease in these markers is a reliable sign of adherence to antiresorptive therapy, and a reduction in fracture risk can be expected.[11]

If association of too low bone turnover with bone fragility seems commonsense, this has not been definitely shown in humans. Low BTMs cannot serve as a warning in individual patients on antiresorptive therapies without thorough clinical judgment.

SUMMARY

As populations age all over the world, the number of osteoporotic fractures will increase. BMD measurement remains the major way to diagnose osteoporosis and to indicate therapy. However, many fractures occur despite T score values higher than −2.5. The FRAX tool, based on clinical risk factors, estimates the 10-year risk of hip and major osteoporotic fractures. The association of BMD and FRAX measurements has improved the identification of patients who are most at risk. It is also possible to update the FRAX tool.[11,12] However, some patients can still be overlooked and denied therapy, albeit probably only a few.[81] Adding the measure of BTMs to the former risk factors and their follow-up during therapy could best address the efficacy of treatment of osteoporosis. However, if their use is of utmost scientific value to understanding the mechanisms of action of new drugs, but may be not for future molecules, it remains to be proved that they are cost-effective in an individual patient in general practice. Moreover, the best BTM to use remains to be determined. The ratio of extra patients found at risk by BTMs to the cost of the BTM measurements is still to be determined.

ACKNOWLEDGMENTS

The authors are grateful to Marie-Christine Hallot for her expert assistance in typing the manuscript.

REFERENCES

1. Mulcahy LE, Taylor D, Lee TC, et al. RANKL and OPG activity is regulated by injury size in networks of osteocyte-like cells. Bone 2011;48:182–8.
2. Parfitt AM. What is the normal rate of bone remodeling? Bone 2004;35:1–3.
3. Glover SJ, Gall M, Schoenborn-Kellenberger O, et al. Establishing a reference interval for bone turnover markers in 637 healthy, young, premenopausal women from United Kingdom, France, Belgium, and the United States. J Bone Miner Res 2009;24:389–97.
4. Recker RR, Kimmel DB, Parfitt AM, et al. Static and tetracycline-based bone histomorphometric data from 34 normal postmenopausal females. J Bone Miner Res 1988;3:133–44.
5. Johnell O, Oden A, De Laet C, et al. Biochemical indices of bone turnover and the assessment of fracture probability. Osteoporos Int 2002;13:523–6.
6. Consensus development conference. Diagnosis, prophylaxis and treatment of osteoporosis. Am J Med 1993;94:646–50.
7. World Health Organization. Assessment of fracture risk and its application to screening for postmenopausal osteoporosis. Technical report – series n 843. Geneva (Switzerland): WHO; 1994.
8. Kanis JA, Devogelaer J-P, Gennari C. Practical guide for the use of bone mineral measurements in the assessment of treatment of osteoporosis: a position paper of the European Foundation for Osteoporosis and Bone Disease. On behalf of the Scientific Advisory Board and the Board of National Societies. Osteoporos Int 1996;6:256–61.
9. Kanis JA, Johnell O, Oden A, et al. FRAX™ and the assessment of fracture probability in men and women from the UK. Osteoporos Int 2008;19:385–97.
10. Marshall D, Johnell O, Wedel H. Meta-analysis of how well measures of bone mineral density predict occurrence of osteoporotic fractures. Br Med J 1996; 312:1254–9.
11. Kanis JA, Johansson H, Oden A, et al. The effects of a FRAX® revision for the USA. Osteoporos Int 2010;21:35–40.
12. Kanis JA, Johansson H, Oden A, et al. Guidance for the adjustment of FRAX according to the dose of glucocorticoids. Osteoporos Int 2011;22:809–16.
13. McClung MR, Geusens P, Miller PD, et al. Effect of risedronate on the risk of hip fracture in elderly women. For the Hip Intervention Program Study Group. N Engl J Med 2001;344:333–40.
14. Siris EC, Chen YT, Abbott TA, et al. Bone mineral density thresholds for pharmacological intervention to prevent fractures. Arch Intern Med 2004;164:1108–12.

15. Garnero P, Sornay-Rendu E, Chapuy MC, et al. Increased bone turnover in late postmenopausal women is a major determinant of osteoporosis. J Bone Miner Res 1996;11:337–49.
16. Devogelaer JP, Depresseux G, Le Thi C, et al. Seasonal variation in bone mineral content in postmenopausal women. In: Dequeker J, Geusens P, Wahner HW, editors. Bone mineral measurement by photon absorptiometry. Leuven (Belgium): Leuven University Press; 1988. p. 225.
17. Rapuri PB, Kinayamu HK, Gallagher JC, et al. Seasonal changes in calciotropic hormones, bone markers, and bone mineral density in elderly women. J Clin Endocrinol Metab 2002;87:2024–32.
18. Storm D, Eslin R, Porter ES, et al. Calcium supplementation prevents seasonal bone loss and changes in biochemical markers of bone turnover in elderly New England women: a randomized placebo-controlled trial. J Clin Endocrinol Metab 1998;83:3817–25.
19. Manios Y, Moschonis G, Trovas G, et al. Changes in biochemical indexes of bone metabolism and bone mineral density after 12-mo dietary intervention program: the postmenopausal health study. Am J Clin Nutr 2007;86:781–9.
20. Bonjour JP, Brandolini-Bunlon M, Boirie Y, et al. Inhibition of none turnover by milk intake in postmenopausal women. Br J Nutr 2008;100:866–74.
21. Macdonald HM, Black AJ, Aucott L, et al. Effect of potassium citrate supplementation or increased fruit and vegetable intake on bone metabolism in healthy postmenopausal women: a randomized controlled trial. Am J Clin Nutr 2008;88:465–74.
22. Macdonald HM, New SA, Golden MH, et al. Nutritional associations with bone loss during the menopausal transition: evidence of a beneficial effect of calcium, alcohol, and fruit and vegetable nutrients and of a detrimental effect of fatty acids. Am J Clin Nutr 2004;79:155–65.
23. Ivaska KK, Gerdhem P, Akesson K, et al. Effect of fracture on bone turnover markers: a longitudinal study comparing marker levels before and after injury in 113 elderly women. J Bone Miner Res 2007;22:1155–64.
24. Marcus R, Holloway L, Wells B, et al. The relationship of biochemical markers of bone turnover to bone density changes in postmenopausal women: results from the Postmenopausal Estrogen/Progestin Interventions (PEPI) trial. J Bone Miner Res 1999;14:1583–95.
25. Chapuy MC, Schott AM, Garnero P, et al. Healthy elderly French women living at home have secondary hyperparathyroidism and high bone turnover in winter (EPIDOS study group). J Clin Endocrinol Metab 1996;81:1129–33.
26. Garnero P, Hausherr E, Chapuy MC, et al. Markers of bone resorption predict hip fracture in elderly women: the EPIDOS prospective study. J Bone Miner Res 1996;11:1531–8.
27. Garnero P, Sornay-Rendu E, Claustrat B, et al. Biochemical markers of bone turnover, endogenous hormones and the risk of fractures in postmenopausal women: the OFELY study. J Bone Miner Res 2000;15:1526–36.
28. Ivaska KK, Gerdhem P, Vaananen HK, et al. Bone turnover markers and prediction of fracture: a prospective follow-up study of 1040 elderly women for a mean of 9 years. J Bone Miner Res 2010;25:393–403.
29. Sornay-Rendu E, Munoz F, Garnero P, et al. Identification of osteopenic women at high risk of fracture: the OFELY study. J Bone Miner Res 2005;20:1813–9.
30. Ross PD, Kress BC, Parson RE, et al. Serum bone alkaline phosphatase and calcaneus bone density predict fractures: a prospective study. Osteoporos Int 2000;11:76–82.

31. Szulc P, Chapuy M-C, Meunier PJ, et al. Serum undercarboxylated osteocalcin is a marker of the risk of hip fracture: a three year follow-up study. Bone 1996;5: 487–8.

32. Vergnaud P, Garnero P, Meunier PJ, et al. Undercarboxylated osteocalcin measured with a specific immunoassay predicts hip fracture in elderly women: the EPIDOS study. J Clin Endocrinol Metab 1997;82:719–24.

33. Chapurlat RD, Garnero P, Breart G, et al. Serum type 1 collagen breakdown products (serum CTX) predicts hip fracture in elderly women: the EPIDOS study. Bone 2000;27:283–6.

34. Szulc P, Montella A, Delmas PD. High bone turnover is associated with accelerated bone loss but not with increased fracture risk in men aged 50 and over: the prospective MINOS study. Ann Rheum Dis 2008;67:1249–55.

35. Chaitou A, Boutroy S, Vilayphiou N, et al. Association between bone turnover rate and bone microarchitecture in men: the STRAMBO study. J Bone Miner Res 2010; 25:2313–23.

36. Alexopoulou O, Jamart J, Devogelaer JP, et al. Bone density and markers of bone remodeling in type 1 male diabetic patients. Diabetes Metab 2006;32:453–8.

37. Ivaska KK, Lenora J, Gerdhem P, et al. Serial assessment of serum bone metabolism markers identifies women with the highest rate of bone loss and osteoporosis risk. J Clin Endocrinol Metab 2008;93:2622–32.

38. Dresner-Pollak R, Parker RA, Poku M, et al. Biochemical markers of bone turnover reflect femoral bone loss in elderly women. Calcif Tissue Int 1996;59:328–33.

39. Ross PD, Knowlton W. Rapid bone loss is associated with increased levels of biochemical markers. J Bone Miner Res 1998;13:297–302.

40. Garnero P, Sornay-Rendu E, Duboeuf F, et al. Markers of bone turnover predict postmenopausal forearm bone loss over 4 years: the OFELY study. J Bone Miner Res 1999;14:1614–21.

41. Hansen MA, Overgaard K, Riis BJ, et al. Role of peak bone mass and bone loss in postmenopausal osteoporosis: 12 year study. Br Med J 1991;303:961–4.

42. Lenora J, Ivaska KK, Obrant KJ, et al. Prediction of bone loss using biochemical markers of bone turnover. Osteoporos Int 2007;18:1297–305.

43. Rogers A, Hannon RA, Eastell R. Biochemical markers as predictors of rates of bone loss after menopause. J Bone Miner Res 2000;15:1398–404.

44. Devogelaer JP, Nagant de Deuxchaisnes C. Use of pamidronate in chronic and acute bone loss conditions. Medicina 1997;57(Suppl 1):101–8.

45. Bauer DC, Garnero P, Hochberg MC, et al. Pretreatment levels of bone turnover and the fracture efficacy of alendronate: the fracture intervention trial. J Bone Miner Res 2006;21:292–9.

46. Seibel MJ, Naganathan V, Barton I, et al. Relationship between pretreatment bone resorption and vertebral fracture incidence in postmenopausal women treated with risedronate. J Bone Miner Res 2004;19:323–9.

47. Bauer DC, Black DM, Garnero P, et al. Change in bone turnover and hip, non-spine, and vertebral fracture in alendronate-treated women: the Fracture Intervention Trial. J Bone Miner Res 2004;19:1250–8.

48. Schousboe JT, Bauer DC, Nyman JA, et al. Potential for bone turnover markers to cost-effectively identify and select post-menopausal osteopenic women at high risk of fracture for bisphosphonate therapy. Osteoporos Int 2007;18:201–10.

49. Chen P, Satterwhite JH, Licata AA, et al. Early changes in biochemical markers of bone formation predict BMD response to teriparatide in postmenopausal women with osteoporosis. J Bone Miner Res 2005;20:962–70.

50. Eastell R, Chen P, Saag KG, et al. Bone formation markers in patients with glucocorticoid-induced osteoporosis treated with teriparatide or alendronate. Bone 2010;46:929–34.
51. Burshell AL, Möricke R, Correa-Rotter R, et al. Correlations between biochemical markers of bone turnover and bone density responses in patients with glucocorticoid-induced osteoporosis treated with teriparatide or alendronate. Bone 2010;46:935–9.
52. Devogelaer JP, Adler RA, Recknor C, et al. Baseline glucocorticoid dose and bone mineral density response with teriparatide or alendronate therapy in patients with glucocorticoid-induced osteoporosis. J Rheumatol 2010;37:141–8.
53. Harris ST, Watts NB, Genant HK, et al. Effects of risedronate treatment on vertebral and non-vertebral fractures in women with postmenopausal osteoporosis: a randomized controlled trial. JAMA 1999;282:1344–52.
54. Eastell R, Barton I, Hannon RA, et al. Relationship of early changes in bone resorption to the reduction in fracture risk with risedronate. J Bone Miner Res 2003;18:1051–6.
55. Delmas PD, Recker RR, Chesnut CH, et al. Daily and intermittent oral ibandronate normalize bone turnover and provide significant reduction in vertebral fracture risk: results from the BONE study. Osteoporos Int 2004;15:792–8.
56. Cummings SR, Karpf DB, Harris F, et al. Improvement in spine bone density and reduction in risk of vertebral fractures during treatment with antiresorptive drugs. Am J Med 2002;112:281–9.
57. Bone HG, Hosking D, Devogelaer JP, et al, Alendronate Phase III Osteoporosis Treatment Study Group. Ten years' experience with alendronate for osteoporosis in postmenopausal women. N Engl J Med 2004;350:1189–99.
58. Glover SJ, Eastell R, McCloskey EV, et al. Rapid and robust response of biochemical markers of bone formation to teriparatide therapy. Bone 2009;45: 1053–8.
59. Heaney RP, Watson P. Variability in the measured response of bone to teriparatide. Osteoporos Int 2010;22(6):1703–8.
60. Zanchetta JR, Bogado CE, Ferretti JL, et al. Effects of teriparatide [recombinant human parathyroid hormone (1–34)] on cortical bone in postmenopausal women with osteoporosis. J Bone Miner Res 2003;18:539–43.
61. Black DM, Greenspan SL, Ensrud KE, et al. The effects of parathyroid hormone and alendronate alone or in combination in postmenopausal osteoporosis. N Engl J Med 2003;349:1207–15.
62. Finkelstein JS, Wyland JJ, Lee H, et al. Effects of teriparatide, alendronate, or both in women with postmenopausal osteoporosis. J Clin Endocrinol Metab 2010;95:1838–45.
63. Meunier PJ, Roux C, Seeman E, et al. The effects of strontium ranelate on the risk of vertebral fracture in women with postmenopausal osteoporosis. N Engl J Med 2004;350:459–68.
64. Bruyere O, Collette J, Rizzoli R, et al. Relationship between 3-month changes in biochemical markers of bone remodelling and changes in bone mineral density and fracture incidence in patients treated with strontium ranelate for 3 years. Osteoporos Int 2010;21:1031–6.
65. Quesada-Gomez JM, Muschitz C, Gomez-Reino J, et al. The effect of PTH (1–84) or strontium ranelate on bone formation markers in postmenopausal women with primary osteoporosis: results of a randomized, open-label clinical trial. Osteoporos Int 2010. [Epub ahead of print].

66. Bjarnason NH, Sarkar S, Duong T, et al. Six and twelve month change in bone turnover are related to reduction in vertebral fracture risk during 3 years of raloxifene treatment in postmenopausal osteoporosis. Osteoporos Int 2001;12: 922–30.
67. Collette J, Bruyere O, Kaufman JM, et al. Vertebral anti-fracture efficacy of strontium ranelate according to pre-treatment bone turnover. Osteoporos Int 2010;21: 233–41.
68. Devogelaer J-P, Boutsen Y, Manicourt DH. Bisphosphonate therapy for the treatment of postmenopausal osteoporosis. Aging Health 2005;1:1–16.
69. Eastell R, Christiansen C, Grauer A, et al. Effects of denosumab on bone turnover markers in postmenopausal osteoporosis. J Bone Miner Res 2011;26:530–7.
70. Delmas PD, Munoz F, Black DM, et al. Effects of yearly zoledronic acid 5 mg on bone turnover markers and relation of PINP with fracture reduction in postmenopausal women with osteoporosis. J Bone Miner Res 2009;24:1544–51.
71. Black DM, Delmas PD, Eastell R, et al. Once-yearly zoledronic acid for treatment of postmenopausal osteoporosis. N Engl J Med 2007;356:1809–22.
72. Cummings SR, San Martin J, McClung MR, et al. Denosumab for prevention of fractures in postmenopausal women with osteoporosis. N Engl J Med 2009; 361:756–65.
73. Bergmann P, Body JJ, Boonen S, et al. Evidence-based guidelines for the use of biochemical markers of bone turnover in the selection and monitoring of bisphosphonate treatment in osteoporosis: a consensus document of the Belgian Bone Club. Int J Clin Pract 2009;63:19–26.
74. Landfeldt E, Ström O, Robbins S, et al. Adherence to treatment of primary osteoporosis and its association to fractures – The Swedish Adherence Register Analysis (SARA). Osteoporos Int 2011. [Epub ahead of print].
75. Delmas PD, Vrijens B, Eastell R, et al. Effects of monitoring bone turnover markers on persistence with risedronate treatment of postmenopausal osteoporosis. J Clin Endocrinol Metab 2007;92:1296–304.
76. Black DM, Schwartz AV, Ensrud KE, et al. Effects of continuing or stopping alendronate after 5 years of treatment: the Fracture Intervention Trial Long-term Extension (FLEX): a randomized trial. JAMA 2006;296:2927–38.
77. Curtis JR, Westfall AO, Cheng H, et al. Risk of hip fracture after bisphosphonate discontinuation: implications for a drug holiday. Osteoporos Int 2008;19:1613–20.
78. Grey A, Bolland MJ, Wattie D, et al. The antiresorptive effects of a single dose of zoledronate persist for two years: a randomized, placebo-controlled trial in osteopenic postmenopausal women. J Clin Endocrinol Metab 2009;94:538–44.
79. Sellmeyer DE. Atypical fractures as a potential complication of long-term bisphosphonate therapy. JAMA 2010;304:1480–4.
80. Marx RE, Cillo JE Jr, Ulloa JJ. Oral bisphosphonate-induced osteonecrosis: risk factors, prediction of risk using serum CTX testing, prevention, and treatment. J Oral Maxillofac Surg 2007;65:2397–410.
81. Hillier TA, Cauley JA, Rizzo JH, et al. The WHO absolute fracture risk models (FRAX): do clinical risk factors improve fracture prediction in older women without osteoporosis? J Bone Miner Res 2011. [Epub ahead of print].

Long-term Safety Concerns of Antiresorptive Therapy

Jie Zhang, PhD[a], Kenneth G. Saag, MD, MSc[b],
Jeffrey R. Curtis, MD, MS, MPH[c],*

KEYWORDS

• Osteoporosis • Anti-resorptive therapy • Safety concerns

Bisphosphonates prevent the loss of bone mineral content by inhibiting bone resorption. As a result, bone turnover is decreased and bone mineral density maintained or even increased. Currently, bisphosphonates account for approximately 80% of all medications prescribed for osteoporosis.[1] Although these medications were well tolerated and safe during large-scale clinical trials, several rare and potentially serious adverse events are reported to be associated with long-term bisphosphonate use from postmarketing reports and epidemiologic studies. These adverse events include osteonecrosis of the jaw (ONJ), atypical fractures, and esophageal cancer. This review summarizes studies examining the association between long-term bisphosphonate use and these adverse outcomes.

BISPHOSPHONATE-RELATED OSTEONECROSIS OF THE JAW
Putative Pathogenesis

ONJ affects the maxilla and the mandible, with the defining symptom of prolonged exposed mandibular and/or maxillary bone, after an insult to the jaw, leading to an

Financial disclosure/conflict of interest: JRC—consulting/honoraria: Amgen, Merck, Novartis, Roche, Lilly; KGS—consulting/honoraria: Amgen, Lilly, Merck, Novartis.
This project was supported by Grant Number T32HS013852 from the Agency for Healthcare Research and Quality (JZ), by Grant Number AR053351 from the National Institutes of Health (JRC), and by Grant Number R01HS018517 from the Agency for Healthcare Research and Quality (JRC). The content is solely the responsibility of the authors and does not necessarily represent the official views of the Agency for Healthcare Research and Quality.
[a] Health Services/Comparative Effectiveness Research Training Program, Department of Epidemiology, University of Alabama at Birmingham, 1665 University Boulevard, RPHB 517B, Birmingham, AL 35294, USA
[b] Division of Clinical Immunology & Rheumatology, University of Alabama at Birmingham, Faculty Office Tower 820, 510 20th Street South, Birmingham, AL 35294, USA
[c] Division of Clinical Immunology & Rheumatology, University of Alabama at Birmingham, Faculty Office Tower 805D, 510 20th Street South, Birmingham, AL 35294, USA
* Corresponding author.
E-mail address: jcurtis@uab.edu

Rheum Dis Clin N Am 37 (2011) 387–400
doi:10.1016/j.rdc.2011.08.001
0889-857X/11/$ – see front matter © 2011 Elsevier Inc. All rights reserved.

rheumatic.theclinics.com

oral lesion with delayed healing. Historically, from the mid-1880s until the 1900s, jaw osteonecrosis, known as phossy jaws, symptomatically resembled ONJ cases associated with bisphosphonate use and was once epidemic among workers of the match industry due to occupational exposure to high level of phosphorous fume.[2] Before ONJ was associated with bisphosphonate use, it was primarily associated with radiation to the head and neck for cancer treatment.

The pathogenesis of so-called bisphosphonate-related ONJ is not clear and has been hypothesized to involve multiple processes. It has been postulated that reduced bone remodeling associated with bisphosphonate use may lead to an increased risk of developing bone necrosis in select patients. Also, the antiangiogenic effects of bisphosphonates may result in a reduction in the blood supply to the region and contribute to poor wound healing. In addition, infection has also been implicated in the pathogenesis of ONJ.[3]

Case Series and Clinical Features of ONJ

Two case series reported in 2003 and 2004 first suggested an association between bisphosphonate use and ONJ.[3–5] Marx[4] described 36 cases of painful exposed bone in the maxilla and/or mandible; all of the cases used bisphosphonates and most of them for cancer treatment (n = 35). They also described several key clinical features of ONJ, including disproportionately affecting the mandibular bone (81%), most cases (78%) developing after dental extraction, and cases refractory to treatment. Similarly, Ruggiero and colleagues[5] conducted a medical record review of 63 ONJ cases. All of their cases had either a history of cancer or osteoporosis and all of them had used bisphosphonate (56 cases were cancer patients exposed to intravenous bisphosphonates). After these case series, many case reports and case series, mainly among cancer patients, of bisphosphonate-associated ONJ were published.[6,7] These reports further characterized ONJ cases and identified several putative risk factors for ONJ, including greater length and cumulative dose of bisphosphonate use; presence of invasive dental procedures, such as extraction and implant; comorbidities; alcohol and tobacco use; and pre-existing periodontal disease. In a majority of ONJ cases, infection was present. Other common symptoms include bone pain, swelling, paresthesia, purulent discharge, and loosening of teeth. A small proportion of these cases were asymptomatic.

Few of these case series included ONJ patients receiving bisphosphonates for osteoporosis but mostly for malignancy. A case series from Italy, including patients with both indications (24 osteoporosis patients and 78 cancer patients), reported that the oral lesions were generally less severe in osteoporosis patients than in cancer patients with bisphosphonate-related ONJ.[8] Another institution-based case series at the University of Southern California identified 9 ONJ cases treated with oral bisphosphonate for osteoporosis. Among these cases, the age ranged from 63 or 80 years and all were preceded by tooth extraction or denture trauma. One significant finding was that the duration of oral bisphosphonate use (70 mg of alendronate per week) in 2 of the 9 ONJ cases was as short as 12 months, suggesting that even short-term exposure could increase the risk of ONJ.[9]

Case Definition of ONJ

The American Academy of Oral and Maxillofacial Surgeons (AAOMS) proposed a definition for bisphosphonate-related ONJ that requires the satisfaction of the following criteria: (1) current or prior use of bisphosphonate, (2) an area of exposed bone within the maxillofacial region without healing for more than 8 weeks, and (3) absence of history of radiation to the jaws.[6] The AAOMS further proposed staging criteria that categorized patients into 1 of 4 stages and recommended stage-specific treatment strategies. The

4 stages were patients with asymptomatic necrotic bone (stage 1); patients with necrotic bone accompanied by infection with or without purulent drainage (stage 2); and patients with necrotic bone accompanied by infection, pain, and at least one of the conditions, including pathologic fractures, extraoral fistula, or osteolysis extending to the inferior border (stage 3).[6]

The case definition of bisphosphonate-associated ONJ developed by the American Society for Bone and Mineral Research (ASBMR) task force was similar except that in cases when the duration of unhealed lesion was less than 8 weeks, the cases should be defined as "suspected" cases and should be followed-up to determine whether they are indeed ONJ cases. To aid the diagnosis of ONJ cases, the task force provided a list of differential diagnosis to be ruled out, such as periodontal disease, gingivitis or mucositis, and infectious osteomyelitis.[7] Such case definition is problematic because the exposure (bisphosphonate use) is part of the case definition.

Epidemiology of ONJ (Frequency of Occurrence)

When discussing the incidence or prevalence of ONJ cases, it is important to define the at-risk population because ONJ has been reported far more frequently in patients treated for cancer than for osteoporosis. Other considerations include the definition of the outcome because surrogate outcomes other than ONJ were used in some studies, and the methods used to define the at risk population and to ascertain ONJ cases were highly variable.

The incidence of ONJ among cancer patients has been estimated to range from 2% to 6%.[10–12] From the database of myeloma patients at the University of Maryland (n = 340), 11 (3% of myeloma patients) ONJ cases were identified.[12] At the University of Texas MD Anderson Cancer Center, a chart review of 3994 patients treated with intravenous bisphosphonate was conducted and 29 ONJ cases were identified among patients with breast cancer (n = 16) and myeloma (n = 13), resulting in incidence proportions of 1.2% and 2.4%, respectively.[10] In a population-based study using linked data from the Surveillance, Epidemiology and End Results (SEER) Program and Medicare, a 6-year cumulative incidence rate of 5.5% for jaw or facial surgery or a diagnosis of inflammatory conditions of osteomyelitis of the jaw was reported among all cancer patients.[11] A limitation of the study was that surrogate outcomes (oral surgery or inflammatory conditions of osteomyelitis of the jaw) were used rather than a clinical ONJ case definition.

The occurrence of ONJ in patients receiving bisphosphonate for osteoporosis is rare. Several epidemiologic studies have generated prevalence estimates ranging from 1 to 20 per 1000.[13–15] In a study conducted in Australia and New Zealand, oral and maxillofacial surgeons in the two countries were surveyed to identify ONJ cases treated with bisphosphonate and the total number of bisphosphonate users estimated using various prescription databases was used as the denominator. When patients treated with bisphosphonates for reasons other than osteoporosis were excluded, there were 36 ONJ cases and the prevalence of ONJ among them was estimated at between 1 and 4 per 1000. The corresponding estimates were 10 times higher among those who had dental extraction.[13] In another study conducted within a large health care plan in the United States, oral bisphosphonate users identified based on pharmacy claims were surveyed with regard to ONJ symptoms. A total of 9 ONJ cases were confirmed and the prevalence of ONJ was estimated at between 5 and 20 per 1000.[14] Finally, in a study conducted by Fellows and colleagues,[15] 6 ONJ cases were ascertained among 21,163 oral bisphosphonate users, resulting in a prevalence of 3 per 1000.

Although rare, ONJ cases may occur in individuals not exposed to bisphosphonate. Among enrollees of two large health maintenance organizations that were part of the

Dental Practice-Based Research Network, ONJ cases were ascertained using a 5-step process that incorporated review of diagnosis and procedure codes, electronic medical records and medical charts, and survey of patients, dentists, and oral surgeons. Among a total of 572,606 eligible enrollees, including those with and without presumed ONJ risk factors, a total of 23 confirmed ONJ cases were identified, resulting in an incidence rate of 0.63 (95% CI, 0.39–1.59) per 100,000 person-years.[15] Of the 23 cases, 6 occurred among oral bisphosphonate user, 2 among intravenous (IV) bisphosphonate users, 12 among cancer patients, 4 among patients with history of head and neck radiation, and 3 among patients free of any risk factors (the categories are not mutually exclusive; other risk factors examined included osteoporosis, osteopenia, diabetes, and immune disorders).[15]

Controlled Studies of the Independent Association Between Oral Bisphosphonate Use and ONJ

The association between oral bisphosphonate use and ONJ has been examined in a few controlled studies, most of them reporting a positive association. Etminan and colleagues[16] conducted a nested case-control study using administrative data from Canada to examine the association between oral bisphosphonate use and nonspecific aseptic osteonecrosis (*International Classification of Diseases, Ninth Revision* [*ICD-9*] code 733.4). A total of 196 cases were identified using *ICD-9* diagnosis code and controls were selected to match the cases on age, calendar time, and length of follow-up. Bisphosphonate use in the previous year before ONJ diagnosis was examined. Both current and past oral bisphosphonate use (alendronate, etidronate, and risedronate) were associated with increased risk of aseptic osteonecrosis (odds ratio [OR] 2.9; 95% CI, 1.7–5.1) for bisphosphonate users compared with nonusers).[16] A limitation of the study was that it was conducted before the *ICD-9* code for ONJ was introduced and, as a result, the cases identified were not site-specific.

The association between bisphosphonate for osteoporosis and ONJ, not a surrogate outcome, was examined in two epidemiologic studies conducted using the Dental Practice-Based Research Networks. In the case-control study, ONJ was defined as exposed necrotic bone in the maxilla or mandible regardless of duration or potential cause in patients without history of facial trauma. Practitioners inside and out of the network were contacted and 308 ONJ cases were identified. Of these ONJ cases, 191 agreed to participate in the study and 573 controls were selected from the same practices from which the cases came. After excluding patients with a history of cancer regardless of the site, bisphosphonate use was associated with ONJ and a dose-response was observed between the magnitude of the association and duration of bisphosphonate use. The OR and 95% CI among those with fewer than 2 years, 2 to 5 years, and more than 5 years of bisphosphonate were 5.2 (1.2–22.5), 11.4 (3.2–40.2), and 26.6 (5.3–133.6).[17] In the cohort study, ONJ cases were defined as exposed necrotic lesion in the maxilla or mandible that were confirmed by manual chart review and were systemically ascertained among enrollees of two large health maintenance organizations. Oral bisphosphonate use and osteoporosis diagnosis were both associated with increased odds of having ONJ ORs of 14.9 and 10.3, respectively.[15] In addition to osteoporosis and oral bisphosphonate use, cancer diagnosis, radiation at head and neck, and glucocorticoid exposure were found to be risk factors of ONJ.

Section Summary

The occurrence of ONJ is rare in the general population. Bisphosphonate use in cancer patients seems associated with a significant increase in the risk of developing ONJ; increasing evidence suggests that bisphosphonate use for osteoporosis may also be associated an increased ONJ risk, although the magnitude of the absolute risk of ONJ in osteoporosis patients is low. Several professional societies, including ASBMR, AAOMS, and the American Dental Association, have made recommendations with regard to patient dental care in patients initiating or receiving bisphosphonate therapy.[18] Both ASBMR and AAOMS recommended that when possible, comprehensive dental examination and invasive dental procedures should be performed before initiating intravenous bisphosphonate therapy for cancer treatment. ASBMR does not specifically recommend such precaution, however, in patients initiating bisphosphonate for osteoporosis or Paget disease.[18]

ATYPICAL SUBTROCHANTERIC AND DIAPHYSEAL FRACTURES
Putative Pathogenesis

Safety concerns that long-term bisphosphonate use may adversely affect the repair of microdamage is not new. At least in theory, bisphosphonate may alter the biomechanical properties of bone matrix via its effect on bone collagen and bone mineralization density distribution, resulting in brittle and stiff bones that could fracture with little trauma. Reduced bone remodeling, coupled with the antiangiogenic effect of bisphosphonates, may further impair the healing of stress fractures, which eventually develop into a complete fracture. The putative mechanisms and preclinical studies suggestive of possible mechanisms have been reviewed elsewhere in detail.[19]

Case Series and Clinical Features of Atypical Subtrochanteric and Diaphyseal Fractures

The case series reported by Odvina and colleagues[20] in 2005 first linked long-term bisphosphonate use with low-energy subtrochanteric and diaphyseal fractures. Among a series of 9 patients who had nonspinal fracture while on long-term alendronate therapy, 3 of them had a fracture at the femoral shaft. After the publication of this case series, Lenart and colleagues,[21] in a letter to *The New England Journal of Medicine*, reported 15 cases of postmenopausal women with low-energy subtrochanteric or diaphyseal fractures. The radiographic features of a transverse or oblique pattern with beaking of the cortex and cortical thickening were present in 10 of these patients and these 10 patients had significantly longer duration of alendronate use (7.3 vs 2.8 years, $P<.0001$). In a similar case series of 17 patients who had low-energy subtrochanteric fractures while on alendronate therapy, similar radiographic features were observed.[22] Yet in another retrospective case series, radiographs of 152 femur fractures were reviewed and 20 were determined to have the defining features of atypical fracture on radiograph. Among the 20 subjects, 15 were receiving alendronate with mean treatment duration of 5 years and 2 were receiving risedronate with mean duration of 3 years. In contrast, only 2 patients were taking alendronate and 1 residronate among the 132 patients without the defining radiographic features.[23]

Several clinical features and potential risk factors associated with increased risk of atypical subtrochanteric and diaphyseal fractures have been suggested by the case series, including concomitant glucocorticoid therapy,[20,23] prodromal pain and discomfort,[22,24] low serum 25-hydroxyvitamin D,[23] increased tendency to be bilateral,[22] delayed fracture healing,[20] and stress reaction.[22]

Case Definition of Atypical Subtrochanteric and Diaphyseal Fractures

A provisional case definition was developed by the ASBMR task force for atypical subtrochanteric and diaphyseal fractures.[19] The case definition includes several major and minor features and to qualify for a case, all major features are required to be present, including occurring anywhere along the femoral diaphysis distal to the less trochanter, no or minimal trauma, transverse or short oblique pattern, noncomminuted, and beaking of the cortex.[19] Examples of the minor features are thickened diaphyseal cortices, prodromal symptoms, and bilateral patterns.[19]

Epidemiology of Subtrochanteric and Diaphyseal Fractures (Frequency of Occurrence)

Currently, the incidence or prevalence of atypical subtrochanteric and femoral shaft fractures is unknown because identification of these fractures requires examination of radiographs to determine the presence or absence of the atypical features (discussed previously). To identify any subtrochanteric or femoral shaft fracture, several studies have used administrative data to examine the frequency of occurrence of these fractures regardless of atypical radiographic features. It was estimated that fractures occurring in this region accounted for approximately 4% to 8% of all hip fractures.[25,26] Wang and Bhattacharyya[25] found that although the overall hip fracture incidence has decreased from 1996 to 2007 for both women and men by 32% and 21%, respectively, the incidence of subtrochanteric fractures remained stable among men and increased among women. In another study in which data from National Hospital Discharge Survey (1996–2006) and Market Scan (2002–2006) were examined, the rates of subtrochanteric and femoral shaft fracture remained unchanged over time.[26] Only a small proportion of these subtrochanteric fractures, however, are likely considered atypical based on radiographic features required for the case definition. For example, in a study in which radiographs for more than 600 femur fractures were reviewed, the characteristic radiographic features of atypical fractures were present only in 102 patients.[27] In another study, using *ICD, Tenth Revision* (*ICD-10*) code, 1271 patients were identified as having sustained a subtrochanteric or femoral shaft fracture. After reviewing the radiographs of 1234 patients, however, only 59 (4.8%) of these fractures were classified as atypical.[28]

Controlled Studies of the Independent Association Between Oral Bisphosphonate Use and Atypical Subtrochanteric or Diaphyseal Fracture

The association between bisphosphonate use and subtrochanteric or diaphyseal fractures was examined in several controlled epidemiologic studies and somewhat conflicting results have been reported. Based on data from the Danish National Hospital Discharge Register and the National Prescription Database, subjects who sustained a typical hip, subtrochanteric, or diaphyseal fracture were identified and the distributions of demographic characteristics, alendronate use in the previous year, and level of trauma associated with the fractures were similar across the 3 groups. Using those data, Abrahamsen and colleagues[29] conducted a cohort study and found that the risks of developing a typical hip, subtrochanteric, or femoral shaft fracture were all elevated among alendronate users to a similar extent. Of particular interest, high adherence was associated with reductions in fractures risk across 3 types of fractures, suggesting that the occurrence of fractures at all 3 locations was potentially driven by underlying osteoporosis. Similarly, no association was found in an investigation using data from 3 large randomized trials of oral alendronate and zoledronate totaling 14,195 women. During follow-up, 12 subtrochanteric and diaphyseal fractures based on radiographic report were identified and no association was found between bisphosphonate use and these fractures (hazard ratios [HRs] and 95% CIs were 1.03 [0.06–1.65], 1.33 [0.12–14.7], and 1.51 [0.25–9.00] for each respective trial).[30] Consistent with the 2 reports, the risks of developing subtrochanteric or diaphyseal fractures were similar (HR 1.0; 95% CI, 0.7–1.5) between bisphosphonate and calcitonin/raloxifene users in a recent cohort study conducted among Medicare beneficiaries with supplemental assistance in Pennsylvania and New Jersey from 1996 to 2006. When the analysis was restricted to those treated with bisphosphonate for longer than 5 years, the estimate suggested a nonsignificantly increased risk (HR 2.02; 95% CI, 0.41–10.00).[31]

In contrast to the studies described above, a significant association between bisphosphonate use and subtrochanteric or diaphyseal fractures has been reported in other controlled observational studies. In a retrospective case-control study, cases consisted of postmenopausal women who had a low-energy subtrochanteric or diaphyseal fracture between 2000 and 2007 and patients with low-energy intertrochanteric or femoral neck fractures during the same time period matched by age, body mass index, and race were selected as controls. Cases were more likely to be bisphosphonate users compared with controls (27% vs 11%). When fractures cases were divided into 2 groups, depending on whether the radiographic features of cortical thickening and beaking of the cortex were present or absent, those with these features were more likely to have used bisphosphonate for longer term (mean duration of bisphosphonate use 7.3 vs 2.8 years).[32] A more recent nested case-control study was conducted using administrative data from Canada.[33] The study found that long-term (≥5 years, adjusted OR 2.74, 95% CI 1.25–6.02) bisphosphonate use was associated with increased risk of subtrochanteric and femoral shaft fracture. The association was not present among those with shorter duration of bisphosphonate use (adjusted OR 0.90; 95% CI, 0.48–1.68) and was increased but not statistically significant among those with 3 to 5 years of medication use (adjusted OR 1.59; 95% CI, 0.80–3.15). When typical femoral neck fracture was examined, a trend in the opposite direction was found that longer duration of bisphosphonate use was associated with decreased fracture risk. As part of the study, the investigators evaluated the validity of the *ICD-10* diagnosis codes and reported a positive predictive value and a sensitivity of 91% and 81% to correctly identify the location of fracture (although not atypical radiographic features) after reviewing a total of 2077 charts.[33] The association between bisphosphonate use and atypical fracture was confirmed yet in another recent population-based study conducted in Sweden. In the study, radiographs from women 55 years of age or older who sustained femur fractures in 2008 were reviewed to ascertain atypical features.[28] The relative risk (RR) of atypical fracture associated with bisphosphonate use was 47.3; however, perhaps more importantly, the increase in absolute risk was only 5 per 10,000 person-years. Of particular interest, the study reported that the risk of atypical fracture decreased rapidly after discontinuation of bisphosphonate therapy in contrast to its long-lasting protective effect. The study estimated that the risk of atypical fracture decreased by 70% annually after discontinuation and that the crude incidence among those who last used bisphosphonate 1 to 2 years ago was 0.1 per 10,000 person-year, only slightly above that among those who never used bisphosphonate (crude incidence 0.09 per 10,000 person-years).

Section Summary

Case reports and series initially suggested an association between bisphosphonate use and atypical subtrochanteric and femoral shaft fractures and led to the identification of unique radiographic features that define these fractures. Despite conflicting results reported from epidemiologic studies, increasing evidence suggests an elevated fracture risk in long-term bisphosphonate users (5 years or more). The magnitude of the association between bisphosphonate use and the occurrence of these fractures, however, remains unclear because many of the population-based epidemiologic studies relied on diagnosis codes (*ICD-9* or *ICD-10*) to identify fracture cases based on the location and not the atypical and more specific radiographic features.[29,31,33] In addition, lack of precision in risk estimates was a major limitation in several of these studies due to the small number of atypical fracture cases identified.[30,31]

With increasing evidence pointing to an association between these atypical fractures and long-term bisphosphonate use of 5 years of more, the US Food and Drug Administration issued a warning regarding the possible risk of atypical subtrochanteric and femoral shaft fractures in patients with long-term bisphosphonate use for the prevention and treatment of osteoporosis. The mandated labeling change affected alendronate, risedronate, ibandronate, and zoledronic acid.

ESOPHAGEAL CANCER
Putative Pathogenesis

Esophageal and gastrointestinal events are the most frequent adverse events that were observed during trials of oral bisphosphonate for osteoporosis. Most of these reports have been nonulcer dyspepsia and reflux type symptoms. More serious esophageal problems have also been described. In a clinical trial of oral preparations of pamidronate for patients with Paget disease, 5 patients receiving two different preparations of oral pamidronate developed erosive esophagitis.[34] A case report of a 59-year-old obese woman developing ulcerative esophagitis within 7 days of initiating oral alendronate for osteoporosis was followed by several case series of 15 patients with alendronate-associated esophagitis.[35–37] In addition, one case report described a 70-year-old man who developed esophageal perforation after 3 months of oral alendronate treatment for glucocorticoid-induced osteoporosis.[38]

Case Series of Esophageal Cancer

Given the biologic plausibility of a causal association between bisphosphonates and esophageal pathology, in a letter to *The New England Journal of Medicine*, a Food and Drug Administration investigator described a total of 23 cases of esophageal cancer after alendronate use received between 1995 and 2008. The median duration of alendronate use to diagnosis was 2.1 years and Barrett esophagus was reported in 1 patient. The same letter described another 31 cases of esophageal cancer reported in Europe and Japan among bisphosphonate users. The median time on bisphosophonate therapy until diagnosis was 1.3 years and Barrett esophagus was reported in 3 patients.[39]

Epidemiology of Esophageal Cancer (Frequency of Occurrence)

Rapid increase in the incidence of esophageal cancer since the 1970s has been observed in a several studies in the United States.[40–42] Although the exact mechanism is not known, this increase was in parallel with the rising prevalence of obesity, which may lead to higher intra-abdominal pressure and reflux disease. Using data from the Surveillance Epidemiology and End Results, Pohl and colleagues[40] estimated that the annual incidence of esophageal cancer increased 7-fold from 3.6 per a million in 1973 to 25.6 per a million 2006. The incidence rates of esophageal cancer were compared among oral bisphosphonate users, users of other anti-osteoporosis medications, and SEER rates. The incidence rate of esophageal cancer was not increased among oral bisphosphonate users compared with those taking other osteoporosis medications (incidence rate ratio [IRR] 0.6; 95% CI, 0.1–4.7) or the SEER rate (IRR, 1.1; 95% CI, 0.3, 4.8).[43]

Controlled Studies of the Association Between Oral Bisphosphonate Use and Esophageal Cancer

Since the case series report, several controlled studies were conducted to assess the association between bisphosphonate use and esophageal and gastric cancer. Using data from Danish national registers, oral bisphosphonate use was found protective of esophageal cancer.[44] These studies were reported, however, in the format of letters to the editor and detailed information regarding methods of the study was not available for evaluation.

Using data from the UK General Practice Research Database, both a matched cohort study and a separate case-control study were conducted to examine the association between bisphosphonate use and esophageal cancer and conflicting results were reported.[45,46] In the matched cohort study, all new users of bisphosphonate were identified; and for each bisphosphonate user, a gender-matched, age-matched, and practiced-matched control was identified regardless of bisphosphonate use. The incidences of esophageal and gastric cancer were compared and bisphosphonate use was not associated with an increased incidence for either cancer type.[45] In addition, no association was found in stratified analyses by cumulative bisphosphonate use and by subtypes of bisphosphonate.[45]

In contrast, a case-control study by Green and colleagues,[46] using the same data source, found increased risk of esophageal cancer among oral bisphosphonate users (RR 1.30; 95% CI, 1.02–1.66). When bisphosphonate users were stratified by number of prescriptions (<9 or ≥10) and by duration of use (≥1 year, 1–3 years, and ≥3 years), increased risk was observed only among those who had 10 or more prescriptions (RR 1.93; 95% CI, 1.37–2.70) and not among those who used 9 prescriptions were less (RR 0.98, 98% CI, 0.66–1.31). A dose-response was observed by duration of use that the RRs were 0.98, 1.12, and 2.24 among those who used for no more than a year, 1 to 3 years, and 3 years or more.[46] The results from these two studies cannot be directly compared due to different study designs (case-control vs matched cohort) and different methods used to ascertain esophageal cancer cases, and dissimilar comparator groups. For example, in the matched-cohort study, bisphosphonate users were eligible to be included in the control cohort and, once included, they were removed from the bisphosphonate cohort.

To further ascertain the independent association between bisphosphonate and esophageal cancer, a cohort of patients with Barrett esophagus was identified from the National Veterans Affairs Databases from the Veterans Affairs from 2000 to 2002.[47] Among these patients, incident esophageal cancer cases were identified and controls were sampled using incident density sampling matching on age and date of diagnosis for Barrett's esophagus at a ratio of 1:6. In this population of mostly men (97%), no association was found between bisphosphonate use and esophageal cancer (adjusted OR 0.92; 95% CI, 0.21–4.15).[47]

Section Summary

The biologic plausibility of a causal association between oral bisphosphonate and esophageal cancer, and several case series have raised further questions about whether long-term bisphosphonate use is associated with increased risk of esophageal cancer. Currently, conflicting results are reported from epidemiologic studies that provide only limited evidence either way. Nevertheless, these reports should prompt physicians to ask patients to report early signs and symptoms of esophageal complications that may merit further investigation or closer surveillance.

RISK VERSUS BENEFIT

Despite the uncertainties regarding the associations between bisphosphonate use and these potential serious adverse events, these events have been highly publicized in popular media and high-profile publications. Furthermore, based on these reports, physicians may be deterred from prescribing bisphosphonates for at least the short-term treatment of osteoporosis, a condition that remains currently undertreated. For example, if it is assumed that the 5-year exposure to bisphosphonates doubled the risk of subtrochanteric and diaphyseal fractures and were associated with a 36%

reduction in the risk of typical hip fractures and that an annual risk of all hip fractures among postmenopausal women was 1%, for every 10,000 patients at high risk of fracture, bisphosphonate use would prevent 108 hip fractures and cause 3 additional subtrochanteric and diaphyseal fractures.[48] This calculation demonstrates that the benefits of bisphosphonate treatment, at least in the short term, outweigh the risks of subtrochanteric and diaphyseal fractures. This analysis, however, is based on imperfect data and uncertainty about the magnitude of the association between bisphosphonate use and these potential adverse outcomes that may increase with cumulative bisphosphonate use.

DRUG HOLIDAY

An important clinical implication of these potential adverse events from long-term bisphosphonate use pertains to the question of what is the optimal length of treatment with these agents. Data on potential bisphosphonates adverse effects also should be coupled with evidence that these agents continue exerting a suppressive effect on bone resorption long after they have been discontinued. Data from extensions to two large clinical trials with up to 10 years of follow-up showed that although long-term treatment with bisphosphonate of up to 10 years continued to yield beneficial effect with regard to bone density, patients who discontinued bisphosphonate continued to experience beneficial effect of up to 5 years.[47,49,50] At the completion of the Fracture Intervention Trial, 1099 participants treated with oral alendronate for 5 years in the trial were further randomized to alendronate or placebo for another 5 years. The study showed that an additional 5 years of treatment was not associated with a significantly decreased risk of nonvertebral fractures (RR 1.00; 95% CI, 0.76–1.32) or morphometric vertebral fractures (RR 0.86; 95% CI, 0.60–1.22). The investigators observed a decreased risk of clinical vertebral fractures (RR 0.45; 95% CI, 0.24–0.85) with an absolute risk reduction of 2.9% over 5 years.[49] In a posthoc analysis, they found that risk reduction for hip fracture was present among those with femoral neck T score less than −2.5.[51] In the 6-year to 10-year extension of another trial of oral alendronate in postmenopausal women with osteoporosis, those who were treated with 20 mg per day for 2 years and 5 mg per day for 3 years were assigned to placebo, and at year 10, the bone mineral density at lumbar spine, trochanter, total hip, and total body remained above baseline level.[50] In addition to the data from the two trials of alendronate, it has been demonstrated that after treatment was discontinued after 3 continuous years of treatment with risedronate, the antifracture effect remained for the fourth year and that those treated had a significant lower incidence of morphometric vertebral fracture rates.[52]

In another study using administrative claims data, among subjects who have used bisphosphonate for 2 years with at least moderate compliance to treatment (medication possession ratio >66%), the risk of a subsequent hip fracture was found to increase approximately one year after discontinuation.[53] No significant difference was observed, however, among those more compliant or with a longer duration of bisphosphonate use, although small numbers limited firm conclusions.[49,51,53] Despite the nonrandomized nature of the data, this study suggested that a short-term drug holiday of approximately 1 year may be safely performed in selected subjects.

SUMMARY

Postmarketing reports have examined the association between several serious adverse events and long-term bisphosphonate use for the prevention and treatment of osteoporosis and raised concerns regarding the long-term safety of this class of antiresorptive medications. Because these adverse events seem to occur infrequently to date, conventional clinical trials are underpowered to provide conclusive evidence with regard to their long-term safety. Several epidemiologic studies have been conducted using large databases from various sources and types. These studies consistently reported an association between intravenous bisphosphonate use for cancer treatment and ONJ. Although conflicting results have been reported regarding the association between bisphosphonate used for osteoporosis and atypical fractures, more recent studies suggested the risk of ONJ and atypical fractures may be increased among long-term users. In contrast to bone and jaw data, the association between bisphosphonate use and esophageal cancer has yielded largely inconsistent results to date.

Atlhough these suspected adverse events can be severe, they occur infrequently. Given the efficacy of bisphosphonates in the reduction of vertebral and nonverterbal fractures, the benefits likely outweigh potential risk over the short term for most patients who require treatment for their osteoporosis. In contrast, the long-term use of these agents and, in particular, the selection of patients at higher risk and potentially with higher bone turnover, is an area of growing research interest and controversy. The case series and controlled epidemiologic studies covered in this review are helpful in alerting physicians to identifying patients perhaps who are at increased risk of developing these serious adverse events (eg, patients with Barrett's esophagus) or precursors to some of these events (ie, prodromal bone pain in the thigh). Because bisphosphonates continue to exert a protective effect a long time after treatment discontinuation and given the potentially elevated risk of developing these adverse outcomes suggested to occur in subjects taking long-term bisphosphonate, physicians may wish to evaluate the risk factors for these serious adverse events in patients who had received 5 years or more bisphosphonate treatment with regard to their fracture risk factors and consider a drug holiday in selected patients with their informed consent. In the future, with increased amount postmarketing surveillance data available, well-designed epidemiologic studies with access to clinical data (eg, x-ray images) will hopefully clarify the magnitude of these associations and whether they are real or spurious. Most importantly, future investigation is needed to provide more information on how to correctly identify those who are at most risk of developing these adverse events among bisphosphonate users and in identifying groups most appropriate to receive these drugs in the shorter term.

REFERENCES

1. Devold HM, Doung GM, Tverdal A, et al. Prescription of anti-osteoporosis drugs during 2004-2007—a nationwide register study in Norway. Eur J Clin Pharmacol 2010;66(3):299–306.
2. Marx RE. Uncovering the cause of "phossy jaw" Circa 1858 to 1906: oral and maxillofacial surgery closed case files-case closed. J Oral Maxillofac Surg 2008;66(11): 2356–63.
3. Pazianas M. Osteonecrosis of the jaw and the role of macrophages. J Natl Cancer Inst 2011;103(3):232–40.
4. Marx RE. Pamidronate (Aredia) and zoledronate (Zometa) induced avascular necrosis of the jaws: a growing epidemic. J Oral Maxillofac Surg 2003;61(9):1115–7.
5. Ruggiero SL, Mehrotra B, Rosenberg TJ, et al. Osteonecrosis of the jaws associated with the use of bisphosphonates: a review of 63 cases. J Oral Maxillofac Surg 2004; 62(5):527–34.
6. Advisory Task Force on Bisphosphonate-Related Ostenonecrosis of the Jaws, American Association of Oral and Maxillofacial Surgeons. American Association

of Oral and Maxillofacial Surgeons position paper on bisphosphonate-related osteonecrosis of the jaws. J Oral Maxillofac Surg 2007;65(3):369–76.

7. Khosla S, Burr D, Cauley J, et al. Bisphosphonate-associated osteonecrosis of the jaw: report of a task force of the American Society for Bone and Mineral Research. J Bone Miner Res 2007;22(10):1479–91.

8. Favia G, Pilolli GP, Maiorano E. Osteonecrosis of the jaw correlated to bisphosphonate therapy in non-oncologic patients: clinicopathological features of 24 patients. J Rheumatol 2009;36(12):2780–7.

9. Sedghizadeh PP, Stanley K, Caligiuri M, et al. Oral bisphosphonate use and the prevalence of osteonecrosis of the jaw: an institutional inquiry. J Am Dent Assoc 2009;140(1):61–6.

10. Hoff AO, Toth BB, Altundag K, et al. Frequency and risk factors associated with osteonecrosis of the jaw in cancer patients treated with intravenous bisphosphonates. J Bone Miner Res 2008;23(6):826–36.

11. Wilkinson GS, Kuo YF, Freeman JL, et al. Intravenous bisphosphonate therapy and inflammatory conditions or surgery of the jaw: a population-based analysis. J Natl Cancer Inst 2007;99(13):1016–24.

12. Badros A, Weikel D, Salama A, et al. Osteonecrosis of the jaw in multiple myeloma patients: clinical features and risk factors. J Clin Oncol 2006;24(6):945–52.

13. Mavrokokki T, Cheng A, Stein B, et al. Nature and frequency of bisphosphonate-associated osteonecrosis of the jaws in Australia. J Oral Maxillofac Surg 2007; 65(3):415–23.

14. Lo JC, O'Ryan FS, Gordon NP, et al. Prevalence of osteonecrosis of the jaw in patients with oral bisphosphonate exposure. J Oral Maxillofac Surg 2010;68(2): 243–53.

15. Fellows JL, Rindal DB, Barasch A, et al. ONJ in two dental practice-based research network regions. J Dent Res 2011;90(4):433–8.

16. Etminan M, Aminzadeh K, Matthew IR, et al. Use of oral bisphosphonates and the risk of aseptic osteonecrosis: a nested case-control study. J Rheumatol 2008; 35(4):691–5.

17. Barasch A, Cunha-Cruz J, Curro FA, et al. Risk factors for osteonecrosis of the jaws: a case-control study from the CONDOR dental PBRN. J Dent Res 2011; 90(4):439–44.

18. Novince CM, Ward BB, McCauley LK. Osteonecrosis of the jaw: an update and review of recommendations. Cells Tissues Organs 2009;189(1–4):275–83.

19. Shane E, Burr D, Ebeling PR, et al. Atypical subtrochanteric and diaphyseal femoral fractures: report of a task force of the American Society for Bone and Mineral Research. J Bone Miner Res 2010;25(11):2267–94.

20. Odvina CV, Zerwekh JE, Rao DS, et al. Severely suppressed bone turnover: a potential complication of alendronate therapy. J Clin Endocrinol Metab 2005; 90(3):1294–301.

21. Lenart BA, Lorich DG, Lane JM. Atypical fractures of the femoral diaphysis in postmenopausal women taking alendronate. N Engl J Med 2008;358(12):1304–6.

22. Kwek EB, Goh SK, Koh JS, et al. An emerging pattern of subtrochanteric stress fractures: a long-term complication of alendronate therapy? Injury Feb 2008; 39(2):224–31.

23. Girgis CM, Sher D, Seibel MJ. Atypical femoral fractures and bisphosphonate use. N Engl J Med 2010;362(19):1848–9.

24. Koh JS, Goh SK, Png MA, et al. Femoral cortical stress lesions in long-term bisphosphonate therapy: a herald of impending fracture? J Orthop Trauma 2010;24(2):75–81.

25. Wang Z, Bhattacharyya T. Trends in incidence of subtrochanteric fragility fractures and bisphosphonate use among the US elderly, 1996-2007. J Bone Miner Res 2011;26(3):553-60.
26. Nieves JW, Bilezikian JP, Lane JM, et al. Fragility fractures of the hip and femur: incidence and patient characteristics. Osteoporos Int 2010;21(3):399-408.
27. Dell R, Greene D, Ott S, et al. A retrospective analysis of all atypical femur fractures seen in a large california HMO from the Years 2007 to 2009. J Bone Miner Res 2010;25(Suppl 1).
28. Schilcher J, Michaelsson K, Aspenberg P. Bisphosphonate use and atypical fractures of the femoral shaft. N Engl J Med 2011;364(18):1728-37.
29. Abrahamsen B, Eiken P, Eastell R. Subtrochanteric and diaphyseal femur fractures in patients treated with alendronate: a register-based national cohort study. J Bone Miner Res 2009;24(6):1095-102.
30. Black DM, Kelly MP, Genant HK, et al. Bisphosphonates and fractures of the subtrochanteric or diaphyseal femur. N Engl J Med 2010;362(19):1761-71.
31. Kim SY, Schneeweiss S, Katz JN, et al. Oral bisphosphonates and risk of subtrochanteric or diaphyseal femur fractures in a population-based cohort. J Bone Miner Res 2010 [Epub ahead of print].
32. Lenart BA, Neviaser AS, Lyman S, et al. Association of low-energy femoral fractures with prolonged bisphosphonate use: a case control study. Osteoporos Int 2009;20(8):1353-62.
33. Park-Wyllie LY, Mamdani MM, Juurlink DN, et al. Bisphosphonate use and the risk of subtrochanteric or femoral shaft fractures in older women. JAMA 2011;305(8):783-9.
34. Lufkin EG, Argueta R, Whitaker MD, et al. Pamidronate: an unrecognized problem in gastrointestinal tolerability. Osteoporos Int 1994;4(6):320-2.
35. Maconi G, Bianchi Porro G. Multiple ulcerative esophagitis caused by alendronate. Am J Gastroenterol 1995;90(10):1889-90.
36. Ribeiro A, DeVault KR, Wolfe JT 3rd, et al. Alendronate-associated esophagitis: endoscopic and pathologic features. Gastrointest Endosc 1998;47(6):525-8.
37. Abraham SC, Cruz-Correa M, Lee LA, et al. Alendronate-associated esophageal injury: pathologic and endoscopic features. Mod Pathol 1999;12(12):1152-7.
38. Famularo G, De Simone C. Fatal esophageal perforation with alendronate. Am J Gastroenterol 2001;96(11):3212-3.
39. Wysowski DK. Reports of esophageal cancer with oral bisphosphonate use. N Engl J Med 2009;360(1):89-90.
40. Pohl H, Sirovich B, Welch HG. Esophageal adenocarcinoma incidence: are we reaching the peak? Cancer Epidemiol Biomarkers Prev 2010;19(6):1468-70.
41. Brown LM, Devesa SS, Chow WH. Incidence of adenocarcinoma of the esophagus among white Americans by sex, stage, and age. J Natl Cancer Inst 2008;100(16):1184-7.
42. Pohl H, Welch HG. The role of overdiagnosis and reclassification in the marked increase of esophageal adenocarcinoma incidence. J Natl Cancer Inst 2005;97(2):142-6.
43. Solomon DH, Patrick A, Brookhart MA. More on reports of esophageal cancer with oral bisphosphonate use. N Engl J Med 2009;360(17):1789-90 [author reply: 1791-2].
44. Abrahamsen B, Eiken P, Eastell R. More on reports of esophageal cancer with oral bisphosphonate use. N Engl J Med 2009;360(17):1789 [author reply: 1791-2].
45. Cardwell CR, Abnet CC, Cantwell MM, et al. Exposure to oral bisphosphonates and risk of esophageal cancer. JAMA 2010;304(6):657-63.

46. Green J, Czanner G, Reeves G, et al. Oral bisphosphonates and risk of cancer of oesophagus, stomach, and colorectum: case-control analysis within a UK primary care cohort. BMJ 2010;341:c4444.
47. Nguyen DM, Schwartz J, Richardson P, et al. Oral bisphosphonate prescriptions and the risk of esophageal adenocarcinoma in patients with Barrett's esophagus. Dig Dis Sci 2010;55(12):3404–7.
48. Rizzoli R, Akesson K, Bouxsein M, et al. Subtrochanteric fractures after long-term treatment with bisphosphonates: a European Society on Clinical and Economic Aspects of Osteoporosis and Osteoarthritis, and International Osteoporosis Foundation Working Group Report. Osteoporos Int 2011;22(2):373–90.
49. Black DM, Schwartz AV, Ensrud KE, et al. Effects of continuing or stopping alendronate after 5 years of treatment: the Fracture Intervention Trial Long-term Extension (FLEX): a randomized trial. JAMA 2006;296(24):2927–38.
50. Bone HG, Hosking D, Devogelaer JP, et al. Ten years' experience with alendronate for osteoporosis in postmenopausal women. N Engl J Med 2004;350(12): 1189–99.
51. Schwartz AV, Bauer DC, Cummings SR, et al. Efficacy of continued alendronate for fractures in women with and without prevalent vertebral fracture: the FLEX trial. J Bone Miner Res 2010;25(5):976–82.
52. Watts NB, Chines A, Olszynski WP, et al. Fracture risk remains reduced one year after discontinuation of risedronate. Osteoporos Int 2008;19(3):365–72.
53. Curtis JR, Westfall AO, Cheng H, et al. Risk of hip fracture after bisphosphonate discontinuation: implications for a drug holiday. Osteoporos Int 2008;19(11): 1613–20.

Osteoporosis in Men: Update 2011

Denise L. Orwig, PhD[a],*, Nancy Chiles, BS[a,b], Mark Jones, BS[a,c],
Marc C. Hochberg, MD, MPH[d]

KEYWORDS

- Osteoporosis • Men • Screening • Treatment
- Bone mineral density

During the past year several review articles have been published on the topic of osteoporosis in men.[1,2] These reviews have highlighted recommendations for measuring bone mineral density (BMD) in older men as a means of screening for osteoporosis, use of the World Health Organization (WHO) Fracture Risk Assessment Tool (FRAX) for predicting the absolute risk of hip and major osteoporotic fractures in men, the frequency of secondary causes of osteoporosis in men, laboratory tests that are useful in evaluating men for these conditions,[3] and newer treatments (ie, zoledronic acid and denosumab) for men with osteoporosis that increase BMD and may reduce the risk of fractures. In addition, new data on the prevalence of low BMD and osteoporosis in men in the United States have been published.[4] Finally, readers are recommended to keep abreast of this broad topic by accessing relevant sections in UpToDate.[5–7]

EPIDEMIOLOGY

Osteoporosis, an asymptomatic disease of low bone mass, has received recognition as a public health problem in men, which is attributable not only to the expected increase in the aging population allowing men more years to experience bone loss, but also to the estimated increase in the consequences of low BMD, particularly the increased risk of suffering a fracture.

Disclosures: Dr Orwig, Ms Chiles, and Mr Jones have nothing to disclose. Dr Hochberg is a consultant to Amgen, Eli Lilly and Co., Genentech/Roche, Merck & Co., Inc and Novartis Pharma AG.
[a] Department of Epidemiology and Public Health, School of Medicine, University of Maryland, 660 West Redwood Street, Suite 200, Baltimore, MD 21201, USA
[b] Doctoral Program in Gerontology, School of Medicine, University of Maryland Baltimore and Baltimore County, 660 West Redwood Street, Suite 200, Baltimore, MD 21201, USA
[c] Epidemiology Doctoral Program, School of Medicine, University of Maryland, 660 West Redwood Street, Suite 200, Baltimore, MD 21201, USA
[d] Department of Medicine, School of Medicine, University of Maryland, 10 South Pine Street, MSTF 8-34, Baltimore, MD 21201, USA
* Corresponding author.
E-mail address: dorwig@epi.umaryland.edu

Rheum Dis Clin N Am 37 (2011) 401–414
doi:10.1016/j.rdc.2011.08.004
0889-857X/11/$ – see front matter © 2011 Elsevier Inc. All rights reserved.

According to the National Osteoporosis Foundation (NOF), 10 million Americans older than 50 years are afflicted with osteoporosis (defined as a BMD less than 2.5 standard deviations below the mean [comprising young normals at peak BMD] or T score <−2.5 SD[8]) and 34 million with low bone mass, or osteopenia (−2.5 SD ≤ T score ≤−1.0 SD).[9] While women are much more likely than men to be diagnosed with osteoporosis and osteopenia,[10] men are also at risk of developing osteoporosis or low bone mass as they age. A more recent methodology for estimating the prevalence of osteoporosis in men applied the NOF guidelines for treatment. These guidelines are based on the WHO FRAX, which estimates a person's 10-year fracture risk based on 10 risk factors.[11] Using these new guidelines, Berry and colleagues[11] found that 17% of men over the age of 50 years met treatment criteria. Dawson-Hughes and colleagues[10] also applied the NOF guidelines to National Health and Nutrition Examination Survey (NHANES) data and found that an estimated 20% of men met the criteria for treatment of low bone mass.

Like women, men have an increasing prevalence of osteoporosis and osteopenia with increasing age; however, the prevalence of osteoporosis is low until 80 years and beyond. NHANES data showed that 27.4% of men aged 50 to 59 years had osteopenia and none had osteoporosis. These percentages rose to 49.1% and 16.6%, respectively, in men older than 80 years.[10] The NOF estimates that the overall prevalence of osteoporosis will increase by almost 50% by the year 2020, when 61.4 million adults in the United States are expected to be affected. The overall prevalence of osteoporosis in men is also expected to increase by 50% in the next 15 years.[12]

The prevalence of osteoporosis differs by race in both genders. White non-Hispanics still have the highest prevalence in both females and males (19%–20% female, 4%–5% male), and among men, non-Hispanic black men (3%) have a slightly higher prevalence than Hispanic men (2%).[10]

Fractures

Having osteoporosis increases the susceptibility to fracture. Approximately 1.5 million fractures a year in the United States are attributable to low bone mass.[13] The most common types of fractures are vertebral, hip, and wrist.[14] The lifetime risk of any fracture for men after the age of 60 years is 25%, and the risk increases to 42% for men diagnosed with osteoporosis.[15] Although diminishing bone strength increases the risk of fracture, the majority of fractures occur in individuals with osteopenia.[16]

The estimated annual cost of fractures in the United States is upwards of $20 billion a year in medical costs.[17] The cost for fractures associated with low bone mass in white men is about $3.2 billion per year.[18] Even though vertebral fractures are the most prevalent of the fragility fractures, hip fractures are the most costly and are associated with the most serious outcomes.

Hip Fractures

In 2004 there were approximately 329,000 hip fractures in the United States and about 28% (93,000) occurred in men.[19] At age 50 years, the lifetime incidence of hip fracture for men is 6% to 11%.[20] Chang and colleagues[21] found that for men the rate increased from zero per 100,000 person years in the 60- to 64-year age group to 1187 per 100,000 person years in the 85 years and older group. Whereas the incidence of hip fracture in women appears to be stabilizing, the incidence in men is on the increase.[22,23] Cummings and colleagues[24] reported from the Study of Osteoporotic Fractures in Men (MrOS) that a lower total hip BMD is associated with an increased risk of hip fracture, and this association is stronger in men than in women despite the higher incidence of hip fractures in women.

Outcomes of Hip Fracture

The consequences of a hip fracture can be severe. In general, men have poorer outcomes after hip fracture than women. Mortality rates are doubled in men.[25,26] In a large study of more than 43,000 veterans, Bass and colleagues[25] found that 32% of men died within a year of fracturing a hip. One explanation for the disparity in mortality rate is that men are often sicker at the time of the fracture than women.[26] Men also have been found to have significantly more postoperative complications than women, which contribute to the increased mortality.[26] Non-Hispanic whites in both genders have been found to have a better survival rate than other races after a hip fracture.[27]

In addition, the risk of suffering a subsequent fracture increases 1.62-fold.[28] Bischoff and colleagues[29] found that in hip fracture patients, 10.3% of participants had a second fracture within 3 years and that men were more likely than women to sustain a second hip fracture (14.4% vs 9.5%). Functional recovery can be lengthy and in some instances, prefracture functional levels are not attained. Of those who were not institutionalized before fracture, 25% remain in an institution a year or longer after fracture, and as many as half of those who were functioning independently before fracture do not recover.[30] Men have poorer function in physical activities in the 12 months after the hip fracture.[25,26,31] In addition, having a diagnosis of osteoporosis can affect men's perception of health. Men with the diagnosis of osteoporosis rated poorer mental health, vitality, and physical functioning according to the SF-36 health questionnaire compared with men without the diagnosis.[32]

RISK FACTORS FOR OSTEOPOROSIS IN MEN
Low Bone Mineral Density

Peak bone mass occurs for most individuals in their early 20s. Factors that influence peak bone mass are genetics, nutrition, exercise, smoking, and alcohol use[33]; however, McGuigan and colleagues[34] found that exercise was the most important predictor for peak bone mass in men. Other significant predictors of peak bone mass in men are weight and alcohol intake.[34] In general, at peak bone mass men have larger bones with greater mass than women.[35]

Gender and race also have an impact on bone loss with age. While men lose bone mass with age,[36] the average rate of bone loss in older men can reach 1% per year.[37,38] In old age, men have lost about one-third of their trabecular bone mass.[39] Studies have found that in both genders, blacks have a slower rate of decline in bone mass than whites.[40,41]

There are several risk factors that appear to be more predictive of developing osteoporosis or osteopenia in men than others. Age, smoking, low body weight, weight loss, positive family history, prior fracture, alcohol use, long-term glucocorticoid use, physical inactivity, and inadequate calcium intake have all been found to be predictive of low bone density in men.[42–45] The MrOS study also reported frailty, falls (factors that contribute to limitations of physical function), and low serum 25-hydroxyvitamin D as risk factors for low BMD in men.[46] Overall, the evidence appears to be strongest for smoking, low body weight, weight loss, age, and long-term glucocorticoid use.[14,42] It is estimated that up to 1 in 6 cases of male osteoporosis is related to glucocorticoid use.[14]

Two additional risk factors have been found to be related to loss of bone mass in men: androgen deprivation therapy for prostate cancer and low testosterone levels.[47–49] Androgen deprivation therapy has been found to decrease bone density in men receiving the treatment at 5 to 10 times the rate of healthy men or those not receiving treatment.[47] The loss is most rapid during the first year of treatment and reverts back to normal age-associated loss after several years.[47,48] Several studies have found that low testosterone levels in older men are also associated with bone loss.[49] The majority of the literature now shows that whereas young men with low testosterone levels are at risk for low bone density, low testosterone levels in older men are not associated with bone loss[14]; rather, it is declining estradiol levels that are more correlated with bone loss in older men.[38,50,51] Two studies found that the men with the greatest risk for hip fracture were those with both low estradiol and low testosterone levels, suggesting there may be a synergistic effect.[2,52,53] It is postulated that the low testosterone levels contribute more to risk factors for falls through muscle mass or balance, and therefore increase the risk of fracture but not risk of low bone density.[2]

Race is also a risk factor for men. Non-Hispanic black men have higher BMD than non-Hispanic white men and Hispanics.[54,55] No evidence has been found that the risk factors for the development of osteoporosis vary within the races. However, there is some evidence that risk factors for fragility fracture vary by race, with androgen deprivation therapy being more of a risk for non-Hispanic white men and age a stronger risk factor for non-Hispanic black men.[16]

DIAGNOSIS AND EVALUATION
Measurement of Bone Mineral Density

The International Society of Clinical Densitometry (ISCD) last updated its official position statement at a Position Development Conference in 2007. The ISCD recommends BMD testing in all men aged 70 years and older, and in men younger than 70 with clinical risk factors for fracture, including a prior history of a fragility fracture, a disease or condition associated with low bone mass or bone loss, and if taking medications associated with low bone mass or bone loss.[56]

BMD should be measured at the lumbar spine and total hip in all subjects. Forearm BMD should only be measured when hip and/or spine cannot be measured or interpreted or when the patient has hyperparathyroidism. A uniform reference database of Caucasian men should be used for calculation of T scores in all ethnic/racial groups. T scores should be used for diagnosis of osteoporosis in men aged 50 years and older; in men younger than 50, osteoporosis cannot be diagnosed solely based on results of BMD testing. The ISCD recommendations have been endorsed by the American Association of Clinical Endocrinologists, the American Society for Bone and Mineral Research, the Endocrine Society, the North American Menopause Society, and the NOF.

The American College of Physicians (ACP) published a clinical practice guideline for screening for osteoporosis in men in 2008.[57] The guideline was based on a systematic literature review commissioned by the Agency for Healthcare Research and Quality.[58,59] The ACP recommended (1) that clinicians periodically perform individualized assessment of risk factors for osteoporosis in older men; and (2) that clinicians obtain dual-energy x-ray absorptiometry (DXA) for men who are at increased risk for osteoporosis and are candidates for drug therapy. Factors that increase the risk for osteoporosis in men include age (>70 years), low body weight (body mass index <20–25 kg/m^2), weight loss (>10% [compared with the usual young or adult weight or weight loss in recent years]), physical inactivity (participates in no physical activities on a regular basis [walking, climbing stairs, carrying weights, housework, or gardening]), corticosteroid use, androgen deprivation therapy, and previous fragility fracture.[58] The US Preventive Services Task Force (PSTF) updated its recommendations in 2010; however, despite evidence in men from longitudinal observational cohort studies that the risk of both vertebral and nonvertebral fractures increases as BMD declines, the PSTF again failed to recommend routine screening of older men for osteoporosis with DXA.[60]

The Department of Veterans Affairs issued an Information Letter in September 2009 concerning osteoporosis in men;[61] this letter was updated in April 2001.[62] It is recommended that an algorithm be used as a guide to choosing which men should be screened for osteoporosis using DXA (**Fig. 1**). Men older than 50 years with any of several underlying conditions are candidates for osteoporosis screening. Examples are men on oral glucocorticoid therapy, those who have already suffered a low-trauma fracture, men treated with androgen deprivation therapy for prostate cancer or anticonvulsants for seizure disorders, and men with malabsorption or alcohol abuse. Men with these and other risk factors need to be considered for bone density testing with DXA.

Evaluation for Secondary Causes

It is estimated that 30% to 60% of osteoporosis in men is secondary,[14] which results from a particular disease or as a result of a medication. Hypogonadism is one such

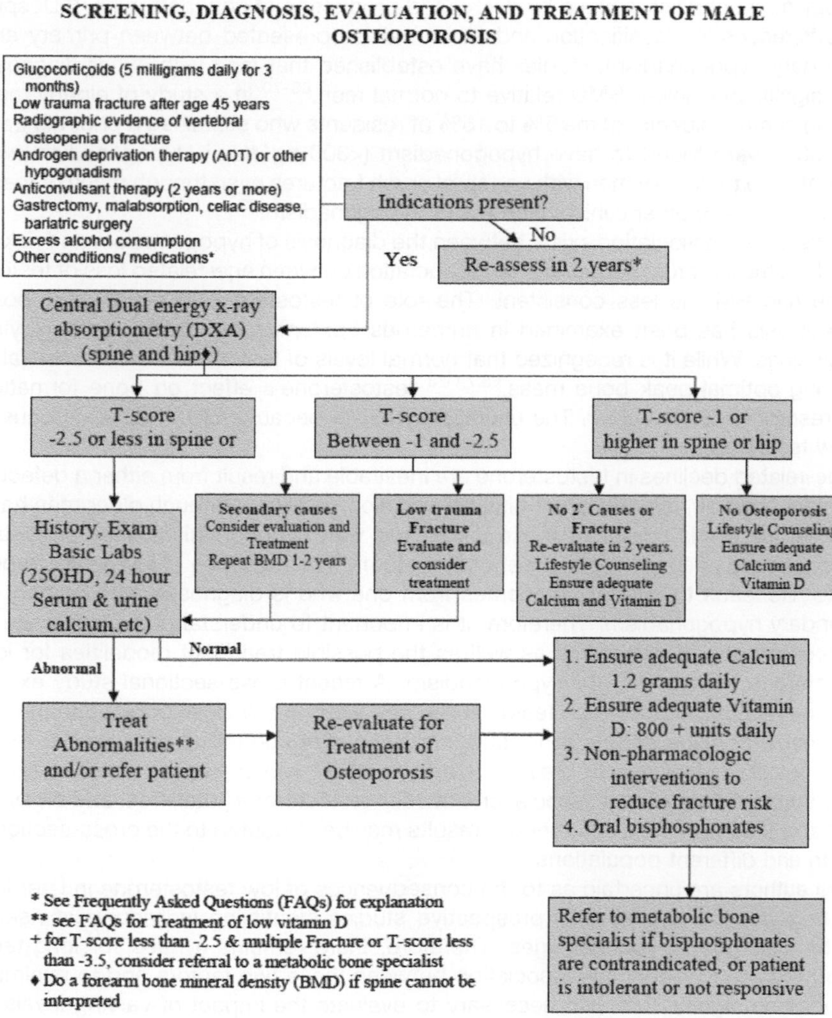

SCREENING, DIAGNOSIS, EVALUATION, AND TREATMENT OF MALE OSTEOPOROSIS

Glucocorticoids (5 milligrams daily for 3 months)
Low trauma fracture after age 45 years
Radiographic evidence of vertebral osteopenia or fracture
Androgen deprivation therapy (ADT) or other hypogonadism
Anticonvulsant therapy (2 years or more)
Gastrectomy, malabsorption, celiac disease, bariatric surgery
Excess alcohol consumption
Other conditions/ medications*

Indications present?
No → Re-assess in 2 years*
Yes

Central Dual energy x-ray absorptiometry (DXA) (spine and hip♦)

T-score -2.5 or less in spine or

T-score Between -1 and -2.5

T-score -1 or higher in spine or hip

History, Exam Basic Labs (25OHD, 24 hour Serum & urine calcium,etc)

Secondary causes Consider evaluation and Treatment Repeat BMD 1-2 years

Low trauma Fracture Evaluate and consider treatment

No 2° Causes or Fracture Re-evaluate in 2 years. Lifestyle Counseling Ensure adequate Calcium and Vitamin D

No Osteoporosis Lifestyle Counseling Ensure adequate Calcium and Vitamin D

Abnormal

Normal

Treat Abnormalities** and/or refer patient

Re-evaluate for Treatment of Osteoporosis

1. Ensure adequate Calcium 1.2 grams daily
2. Ensure adequate Vitamin D: 800 + units daily
3. Non-pharmacologic interventions to reduce fracture risk
4. Oral bisphosphonates

* See Frequently Asked Questions (FAQs) for explanation
** see FAQs for Treatment of low vitamin D
+ for T-score less than -2.5 & multiple Fracture or T-score less than -3.5, consider referral to a metabolic bone specialist
♦ Do a forearm bone mineral density (BMD) if spine cannot be interpreted

Refer to metabolic bone specialist if bisphosphonates are contraindicated, or patient is intolerant or not responsive

Fig. 1.

secondary cause and it is the failure of the testes to produce androgen, sperm, or both. The prevalence of hypogonadism is uncertain, although the results of one study found that prevalence varies across age groups, from 7% of men aged 40 to 60 years, 22% of men 60 to 80 years, and 36% of men 80 to 100 years.[63] Apparent decline in total testosterone in these individuals is compounded in frequency by permanent disorders of the hypothalamic-pituitary-gonadal axis.

Classification of primary or secondary hypogonadism is determined based on the location of the abnormality on the hypothalamic-pituitary-testicular axis. Those with primary hypogonadism have low testosterone, high luteinizing hormone, and high follicle-stimulating hormone levels. The major causes of primary hypogonadism include genetic causes such as Klinefelter syndrome, congenital causes such as anorchia, toxins including alcohol and heavy metals, orchitis, trauma, infarction, and aging.[64] A diagnosis of secondary hypogonadism means that an individual has low testosterone, low luteinizing hormone, and low follicle-stimulating hormone levels. The major causes of secondary hypogonadism include pubertal delay and hypogonadotropism, a condition caused by decreased production of gonadotropins.[64] Despite the differences in classification and abnormalities presented between primary and secondary hypogonadism, studies have established that men with either diagnosis have significantly lower BMD relative to normal men.[65-70] In a study of elderly male nursing home residents, of the 5% to 15% of residents who sustained a prior hip fracture, 66% were found to have hypogonadism (<300 ng/dL).[71] Hypogonadism was present in up to 20% of men with vertebral crush fractures even though many of these men did not have other clinical features of hypogonadism.[72]

While a clear association exists between the diagnosis of hypogonadism and risk of low BMD, the literature supporting the association between age-related loss of testosterone and BMD is less consistent. The role of testosterone in maintaining bone homeostasis has been examined in numerous epidemiologic studies with varying conclusions. While it is recognized that normal levels of testosterone are essential in attaining optimal peak bone mass,[65,73-76] testosterone's effect on bone formation and resorption is less clear. The uncertainty exists because of the different causes of low testosterone.

Age-related declines in testosterone are inevitable and result from either a defect in testicular function, hypothalamic-pituitary function, or both. Although older men have testosterone levels similar to those diagnosed with hypogonadism, they represent a special case due to the late onset of symptoms. The presence of low testosterone in later life leads to different outcomes from one who is diagnosed with primary or secondary hypogonadism. Therefore, it is important to understand the difference in the presentation of symptoms as well as the possible treatment modalities for low testosterone independent of hypogonadism. A recent cross-sectional study examining the relationship between testosterone and BMD in a diverse population of men was unable to discover any significant correlation after controlling for age (utd, 43).[77] These results coincide with previous studies.[78-86] However, results from the MrOS study suggest a significant association between testosterone (total, free, and bioavailable) and BMD.[87-89] The difference in results may be attributed to the cross-sectional design and different populations.

The authors are uncertain as to the consequences of low testosterone in later life, due to a paucity of long-term prospective studies identifying individuals at risk of low testosterone at younger ages. Therefore, there remains a need for long-term cohort studies to clarify the association between these two factors and to minimize temporal ambiguity. It is also necessary to evaluate the impact of varying levels of low testosterone as opposed to no testosterone, such as is found with castrated men, to fully understand the impact of testosterone on BMD.

TREATMENT OF OSTEOPOROSIS IN MEN

Treatment options for osteoporosis include lifestyle modification including calcium and vitamin D supplementation, weight-bearing exercise, smoking cessation and reduction in alcohol intake as well as prescription medications. According to the Institute of Medicine, the recommended dietary allowance for men aged 70 and above for calcium is 1,200 mg per day while that for vitamin D is 800 International Units (IU) per day.

The major class of prescription drugs used in the treatment of osteoporosis in men is bisphosphonates. Three of these are approved by the U.S. Food and Drug Administration (FDA) for treatment of osteoporosis in men: alendronate, risedronate, and zoledronic acid.[2] Alendronate and risedronate are both administered as oral medications while zoledronic acid is administered as an intravenous (IV) infusion. Alendronate should be given at a dose of either 70 mg once weekly or 10 mg daily. Risedronate should be given at a dose of 35 mg once weekly; note that the 150 mg once monthly dose is not FDA approved for use in men. Zoledronic acid should be given at a dose of 5 mg once yearly by IV infusion; it is particularly useful for the patient who is unable to sit or stand upright for at least 30 minutes or with a disorder of the esophagus that impedes swallowing and complete esophageal emptying. All bisphosphonates are contraindicated in patients with hypocalcemia.

Teriparatide, recombinant human parathyroid hormone 1-34, is also approved for treatment of osteoporosis in men; it should be given at a dose of 20 mcg daily as a subcutaneous injection. Teriparatide is indicated in men with primary or hypogonadal osteoporosis at high risk of fracture. In our opinion, it should be reserved for patients who have contraindications to or are intolerant of bisphosphonates, or are considered to have failed bisphosphonate therapy. At this time, denosumab is not yet approved for treatment of osteoporosis in men. We recommend that all health care providers read the Product Information for each compound in order to familiarize themselves with the contraindications, warnings and precautions, adverse reactions and drug interactions for each compound as well as the section on Patient Counseling Information.

The detection and treatment of osteoporosis has been found to be cost-effective and lower mortality in both women and men.[90–93] NOF recommends that men aged 50 years and above with either (1) a hip or vertebral fracture, (2) osteoporosis based on BMD testing (T-score of -2.5 or below at either the lumbar spine or femoral neck, or (3) low BMD (T-score between -1.0 and -2.5) and a 10-year probability of fracture of >20 percent for major osteoporotic fractures or >3 percent for hip fracture be treated with pharmacologic agents to reduce their fracture risk.[94]

In spite of the evidence that men are at risk for low bone mass and fractures, there is a gap in care that exists. Men and racial minorities are less likely to be treated for low bone mass post-fracture than non-Hispanic white women.[95–97] Currently no state or federal coverage for screening or education about osteoporosis exists for men.[9]

As previously mentioned, low serum testosterone may be a risk factor for low BMD and osteoporosis. As a result of this association, testosterone has been used as a possible treatment for low BMD and osteoporosis. Testosterone therapy should provide physiologic range serum testosterone levels (280–800 ng/dL) and physiologic range dihydrotestosterone and estradiol levels.[98] These testosterone levels have been successful in providing optimal virilization and normal sexual function for men.[98]

Some clinical trials that have been performed to test the efficacy of testosterone treatment for low BMD have shown efficacy. In adolescent male patients with hypogonadotropic (primary) hypogonadism, testosterone therapy increased BMD in comparison with that in male patients with hypogonadism not receiving testosterone.[72,99] In men with prepubertal-onset hypogonadotropic hypogonadism, however, diminished bone mass may be only marginally improved by testosterone replacement.[100] The number of studies that have analyzed the effect of testosterone therapy on BMD levels in older men is limited.

Clinical trials performed to identify whether or not testosterone replacement therapy is beneficial in increasing BMD, and reducing fracture risk and rate of bone loss have been limited in sample size and design, as many trials have not utilized a randomized design.[2,7] In addition to improved study characteristics, contraindications for testosterone therapy need to be considered. Hormone therapy may be contraindicated by age. While no limit has been definitively established, it is possible that this contraindication exists for men older than 80 years old.[64] Other contraindications for testosterone therapy include the presence of prostate cancer, male breast cancer, and untreated prolactinoma, as treatment for these diseases can stimulate tumor growth in androgen-dependent neoplasm.[98] Further understanding of the contraindications and risks of testosterone treatment should be evaluated before this treatment is advised for the overall male, low-testosterone population.

Glucocorticoid-induced Osteoporosis

The man with glucocorticoid-induced osteoporosis (GIOP) presents a special problem, particularly for the rheumatologist. Adler and Hochberg recently reviewed the pathophysiology of GIOP and the evaluation and management of men receiving glucocorticoid therapy.[101] The American College of Rheumatology revised its recommendations for the prevention and management of men aged 50 and above with GIOP in 2010.[102] Men are stratified on risk to either a low, medium or high risk group. High risk is defined in men as a BMD T-score of -2.5 or below or a 10-year risk of major osteoporotic fracture greater than 20% using the FRAX algorithm. Medium risk is defined in men as a 10-year risk of major osteoporotic fracture between 10 and 20% with a BMD T-score between -1 and -2.5 (except in Caucasian men aged 80 and above wherein the BMD T-score can be as high as -0.5); and low risk is defined in men as a 10-year risk of major osteoporotic fracture less than 10%. All men at either medium or high risk should receive pharmacologic therapy in addition to calcium and vitamin D supplementation and lifestyle modification. For men at low risk, pharmacologic therapy is recommended only for those receiving daily glucocorticoid doses of 7.5 mg or above prednisone equivalent. Men below the age of 50 years are treated with pharmacologic therapy only if they have a prevalent fragility fracture. Finally, men receiving glucocorticoids who have low serum testosterone levels should be considered for testosterone therapy, in the absence of contraindications, as data suggest that testosterone replacement increases BMD.[103]

REFERENCES

1. Adler RA. Osteoporosis in men: what has changed? Curr Osteoporos Rep 2011; 9(1):31–5.
2. Khosla S. Update in male osteoporosis. J Clin Endocrinol Metab 2010;95:3–10.
3. Ryan C, Petkov VI, Adler RA. Osteoporosis in men: the value of laboratory testing. Osteoporos Int 2011;22(6):1845–53.

4. Looker AC, Melton LJ III, Harris TB, et al. Prevalence and trends in low femur bone density among older US adults: NHANES 2005-2006 compared with NHANES III. J Bone Miner Res 2010;25:64–71.

5. Finkelstein JS. Epidemiology and etiology of osteoporosis in men. UpToDate; 2010. Available at: http://www.uptodate.com. Accessed December 28, 2010.

6. Finkelstein JS. Diagnosis and evaluation of osteoporosis in men. UpToDate; 2010. Available at: http://www.uptodate.com. Accessed December 28, 2010.

7. Finkelstein JS. Treatment of osteoporosis in men. UpToDate; 2010. Available at: http://www.uptodate.com. Accessed December 28, 2010.

8. World Health Organization. Assessment of fracture risk and application to screening for postmenopausal osteoporosis. Geneva (Switzerland): World Health Organization; 1994.

9. National Osteoporosis Foundation. America's bone health: the state of osteoporosis and low bone mass. Available at: http://www.nof.org/advocacy/prevalence. Accessed May 1, 2005.

10. Dawson-Hughes B, Looker AC, Tosteson NA, et al. The potential impact of new National Osteoporosis Foundation guidance on treatment patterns. Osteoporos Int 2010;21:41–52.

11. Berry S, Kiel DP, Donaldson MG, et al. Application of the National Osteoporosis Foundation Guidelines to postmenopausal women and men: the Framingham Osteoporosis Study. Osteoporos Int 2010;21:53–60.

12. Morris C, Cabral D, Cheng H, et al. Patterns of bone mineral density testing: current guidelines, testing, rates, and interventions. J Gen Intern Med 2004; 19(7):783–90.

13. Centers for Medicare and Medicaid Services. Bone Mass Measurement: Overview. 2011. Available at: http://www.cms.gov/BoneMassMeasurement/. Accessed August 10, 2011.

14. Lane J, Serota AC, Raphael B. Osteoporosis: differences and similarities in male and female patients. Orthop Clin North Am 2006;37:601–9.

15. Nguyen N, Ahlborg HG, Center JR, et al. Residual lifetime risk of fractures in women and men. J Bone Miner Res 2007;22(6):781–8.

16. Thomas-John M, Codd MB, Manne S, et al. Risk factors for the development of osteoporosis and osteoporotic fractures among older men. J Rheumatol 2009; 36(9):1947–52.

17. Burge R, Dawson-Hughes B, Solomon DH, et al. Incidence and economic burden of osteoporosis-related fractures in the United States. J Bone Miner Res 2007;22:465–75.

18. Ray NF, Chan JK, Thamer M, et al. Medical expenditures for the treatment of osteoporotic fractures in the United States in 1995: report from the National Osteoporosis Foundation. J Bone Miner Res 1997;12:24–35.

19. DeFrances CJ, Podgornik MN. 2004 National Hospital Discharge Survey: Annual Summary with detailed diagnosis and procedure data. Advance data from vital and health statistics. Hyattsville (MD): National Center for Health Statistics; 2006. Available at: http://www.cdc.gov/nchs/data/ad/ad371.pdf. Accessed August 10, 2011.

20. Melton L III, Orwoll E, Wasnich R. Does bone density predict fractures comparably in men and women? Osteoporos Int 2001;12:707–9.

21. Chang KP, Center JR, Nguyen TV, et al. Incidence of hip and other osteoporotic fractures in elderly men and women: Dubbo Osteoporosis Epidemiology Study. J Bone Miner Res 2004;19(4):532–6.

22. Haentjens P, Johnell O, Kanis JA, et al. Evidence from data searches and life-table analyses for gender-related differences in absolute risk of hip fracture after Colles' or spine fracture: Colles' fracture as an early and sensitive marker of skeletal fragility in white men. J Bone Miner Res 2004;19(12): 1933–44.

23. Melton LJ 3rd, Kearns AE, Atkinson EJ, et al. Secular trends in hip fracture incidence and recurrence. Osteoporos Int 2008;20(5):687–94.

24. Cummings SR. BMD and risk of hip and nonvertebral fractures in older men: a prospective study and comparison with older women. J Bone Miner Res 2006;21(10):1550.

25. Bass E, French DD, Bradham DD, et al. Risk-adjusted mortality rates of elderly veterans with hip fractures. Ann Epidemiol 2007;17(7):514–9.

26. Endo Y, Aharonoff GB, Zuckerman JD, et al. Gender differences in patients with hip fracture: a greater risk of morbidity and mortality in men. J Orthop Trauma 2005;19(1):29–35.

27. Penrod J, Litke A, Hawkes WG, et al. The association of race, gender, and comorbidity with mortality and function after hip fracture. J Gerontol A Biol Sci Med Sci 2008;63A(8):867–72.

28. Colon-Emeric C, Kuchibhatla M, Pieper C, et al. The contribution of hip fracture to risk of subsequent fractures: data from two longitudinal studies. Osteoporos Int 2003;14(11):879–83.

29. Bischoff HA, Solomon DH, Dawson-Hughes B, et al. Repeat hip fractures in a population-based sample of Medicare recipients in the US: timing and gender differences [abstract]. J Bone Miner Res 2001;16(Suppl 1). S213.

30. Magaziner J, Lydick E, Hawkes W, et al. Excess mortality attributable to hip fracture in white women aged 70 years and older. Am J Public Health 1997;87: 1630–6.

31. Hawkes WG, Wehren L, Orwig D, et al. Gender differences in functioning after hip fracture. J Gerontol A Biol Sci Med Sci 2006;61A(5):495–9.

32. Dennison E, Jameson KA, Syddall HE, et al. Bone health and deterioration in quality of life among participants from the Hertfordshire Cohort Study. Osteoporos Int 2010;21(11):1817–24.

33. Heaney RP, Abrams S, Dawson-Hughes B, et al. Peak bone mass. Osteoporos Int 2000;11:985–1009.

34. McGuigan F, Murray L, Gallagher A, et al. Genetic and environmental determinants of peak bone mass in young men and women. J Bone Miner Res 2002; 17(7):1273–9.

35. Cummings SR. Bone biology, epidemiology, and general principles. In: Cummings SR, Cosman F, Jamal S, editors. Osteoporosis: an Evidence-based Guide to Prevention and Management. Philadelphia (PA): American College of Physicians; 2002. p. 3–25.

36. Seeman E, Delmas PD. Bone quality – the material and structural basis of bone strength and fragility. New Engl J Med 2006;354(21):2250–61.

37. Hannan MT, Felson DT, Dawson-Hughes B, et al. Risk factors for longitudinal bone loss in elderly men and women: the Framingham Osteoporosis Study. J Bone Miner Res 2000;15:710–20.

38. Amin S. Male osteoporosis: epidemiology and pathophysiology. Curr Osteoporos Rep 2003;1:71–7.

39. Riggs B, Khosla S, Melton LJ 3rd. Sex steroids and the construction and conservation of the adult skeleton. Endocr Rev 2002;23(3):279–302.

40. Cauley J, Lui LY, Stone KL, et al. Longitudinal study of changes in hip bone mineral density in Caucasian and African-American women. J Am Geriatr Soc 2005;53(2):183–9.
41. Tracy JK, Meyer WA, Flores RH, et al. Racial differences in rate of decline in bone mass in older men: the Baltimore Men's Osteoporosis Study. J Bone Miner Res 2005;20(7):1228–34.
42. Papaioannou A, Kennedy CC, Cranney A, et al. Risk factors for low BMD in healthy men age 50 years or older: a systematic review. Osteoporos Int 2009; 20(4):507–18.
43. Naves M, Diaz-Lopez JG, Gomez C, et al. Prevalence of osteoporosis in men and determinants of changes in bone mass in a non-selected Spanish population. Osteoporos Int 2005;16:603–9.
44. Bakhireva L, Barrett-Connonr E, Kritz-Silverstein D, et al. Modifiable predictors of bone loss in older men: a prospective study. Am J Prev Med 2004;26(5):436–42.
45. Scholtissen S, Guillemin F, Bruyere O, et al. Assessment of determinants for osteoporosis in elderly men. Osteoporos Int 2009;20:1157–66.
46. Lewis C. Predictors of non-spine fracture in elderly men: the MrOS Study. J Bone Miner Res 2007;22(2):211.
47. Greenspan S, Coates P, Sereika SM, et al. Bone loss after initiation of androgen deprivation therapy in patients with prostate cancer. J Clin Endocrinol Metab 2005;90(12):6410–7.
48. Campion J, Maricic MJ. Osteoporosis in men. 2003. Available at: http://www. aafp.org/afp/2003/0401/p1521.html. Accessed August 10, 2011.
49. Meier C, Nguyen TV, Handelsman DJ, et al. Endogenous sex hormones and incident fracture risk in older men. The Dubbo Osteoporosis Epidemiology Study. Arch Intern Med 2008;168(1):47–54.
50. Falahati-Nini A, Riggs BL, Atkinson EJ, et al. Relative contributions of testosterone and estrogen in regulating bone resorption and formation in normal elderly men. J Clin Invest 2000;106:1553–60.
51. Venken K, Callewaert F, Boonen S, et al. Sex hormones, their receptors, and bone health. Osteoporos Int 2008;19(11):1517–25.
52. Amin S, Zhang Y, Felson DT, et al. Estradiol, testosterone, and the risk for hip fracture in elderly men from the Framingham Study. Am J Med 2006;119:426–33.
53. LeBlanc E, Nielson CM, Marshall LM, et al. The effects of serum testosterone, estradiol, and sex hormone binding globulin levels on fracture risk in older men. J Clin Endocrinol Metab 2009;94:3337–46.
54. George A, Tracy JK, Meyer WA, et al. Racial differences in bone mineral density in older men. J Bone Miner Res 2003;18(12):2238–44.
55. Chiu G, Araujo AB, Travison TG, et al. Relative contributions of multiple determinants to bone mineral density in men. Osteoporos Int 2009;20:2035–47.
56. Baim S, Binkley N, Bilezikian JP, et al. Official Positions of the International Society for Clinical Densitometry and executive summary of the 2007 ISCD Position Development Conference. J Clin Densitom 2008;11(1):75–91.
57. Qaseem A, Snow V, Shekelle P, et al. Clinical Efficacy Assessment Subcommittee of the American College of Physicians. Screening for osteoporosis in men: a clinical practice guideline Screening for osteoporosis in men: a clinical practice guideline from the American College of Physicians. Ann Intern Med 2008;148(9):680–4.
58. Shekelle P, Munjas B, Liu H, et al. Screening men for osteoporosis: who & how. Available at: http://www.ncbi.nlm.nih.gov/books/NBK49063/. Accessed August 9, 2011.

59. Liu H, Paige NM, Goldzweig CL, et al. Screening for osteoporosis in men: a systematic review for an American College of Physicians Guideline. Ann Intern Med 2008;148(9):685–701.

60. Nelson HD, Haney EM, Chou R, et al. Screening for osteoporosis: Systematic Review to Update the 2002 U.S. Preventive Services Task Force Recommendation. 2010. Available at: http://www.ncbi.nlm.nih.gov/books/NBK45201/. Accessed August 9, 2011.

61. Department of Veterans Affairs VHA. 2009. Available at: http://www.va.gov/vhapublications/ViewPublication.asp?pub_ID=2083. Accessed August 9, 2011.

62. Petzel RA. Undersecretary for Health's Information Letter. Osteoporosis in Men. Washington, DC: Department of Veterans Affairs, Veterans Health Administration; 2011.

63. Vermeulen A, Kaufman JM. Ageing of the hypothalamo-pituitary-testicular axis in men. Horm Res 1995;43(1–3):25–8.

64. Faiman C. Male Hypogonadism. 2009. Available at: http://www.clevelandclinicmeded.com/medicalpubs/diseasemanagement/endocrinology/male-hypogonadism/. Accessed August 9, 2011.

65. Finkelstein J, Klibanski A, Neer RM, et al. Osteoporosis in men with idiopathic hypogonadotropic hypogonadism. Ann Intern Med 1987;106(3):354–61.

66. Stoch S, Parker RA, Chen L, et al. Bone loss in men with prostate cancer treated with gonadotropin-releasing hormone agonists. J Clin Endocrinol Metab 2001; 86(6):2787–91.

67. Diamond T, Stiel D, Posen S. Osteoporosis in hemochromatosis: iron excess, gonadal deficiency, or other factors? Ann Intern Med 1989;110(6):430–6.

68. Katznelson L, Finkelstein JS, Schoenfeld DA, et al. Increase in bone density and lean body mass during testosterone administration in men with acquired hypogonadism. J Clin Endocrinol Metab 1996;81:4358–65.

69. Behre H, Kliesch S, Leifke E, et al. Long-term effect of testosterone therapy on bone mineral density in hypogonadal men. J Clin Endocrinol Metab 1997;82(8): 2386–90.

70. Finkelstein J, Klibanski A, Neer RM, et al. Increases in bone density during treatment of men with idiopathic hypogonadotropic hypogonadism. J Clin Endocrinol Metab 1989;69(4):776–83.

71. Abbasi A, Rudman D, Wilson CR, et al. Observations on nursing home residents with a history of hip fracture. Am J Med Sci 1995;310(6):229–34.

72. Scane A, Sutcliffe AM, Francis RM. Osteoporosis in men. Bailliere's Clin Rheumatol 1993;7:589–601.

73. Guo C, Jones TH, Eastell R. Treatment of isolated hypogonadotropic hypogonadism effect on bone mineral density and bone turnover. J Clin Endocrinol Metab 1997;82(2):658–65.

74. Finkelstein J, Neer RM, Biller BM, et al. Osteopenia in men with a history of delayed puberty. N Engl J Med 1992;326(9):600–4.

75. Finkelstein J, Klibanski A, Neer RM. A longitudinal evaluation of bone mineral density in adult men with histories of delayed puberty. J Clin Endocrinol Metab 1996;81(3):1152–5.

76. Bertelloni S, Baroncelli GI, Battini R, et al. Short-term effect of testosterone treatment on reduced bone density in boys with constitutional delay of puberty. J Bone Miner Res 1995;10(10):1488–95.

77. Araujo AB, Travison TG, Harris SS, et al. Race/ethnic differences in bone mineral density in men. Osteoporos Int 2007;18(7):943–53.

78. Slemenda C, Longcope C, Zhou L, et al. Sex steroids and bone mass in older men: positive associations with serum estrogens and negative associations with androgens. J Clin Invest 1997;100:1755–9.

79. Khosla S, Melton LJ 3rd, Atkinson EJ, et al. Relationship of serum sex steroid levels and bone turnover markers with bone mineral denstiy in men and women: a key role for bioavailable estrogen. J Clin Endocrinol Metab 1998;83(7):2266–74.

80. Ongphiphadhanakul B, Rajatanavin R, Chanprasertyothin S, et al. Serum oestradiol and oestrogen-receptor gene polymorphism are associated with bone mineral density independently of serum testosterone in normal males. Clin Endocrinol 1998;49:803–9.

81. Center J, Nguyen TV, Sambrook PN, et al. Hormonal and biochemical parameters in the determination of osteoporosis in elderly men. J Clin Endocrinol Metab 1999;84(10):3626–35.

82. Greendale G, Edelstein S, Barrett-Connor E. Endogenous sex steroids and bone mineral density in older women and men: the Rancho Bernardo Study. J Bone Miner Res 1997;12(11):1833–43.

83. Amin S, Zhang Y, Sawin CT, et al. Association of hypogonadism and estradiol levels with bone mineral density in elderly men from the Framingham Study. Ann Intern Med 2000;133(12):951–63.

84. Araujo A, Travison TG, Leder BZ, et al. Correlations between serum testosterone, estradiol, and sex hormone-binding globulin and bone mineral density in a diverse sample of men. J Clin Endocrinol Metab 2008;93(6):2135–41.

85. Meier D, Orwoll ES, Keenan EJ, et al. Marked decline in trabecular bone mineral content in healthy men with age: lack of association with sex steroid levels. J Am Geriatr Soc 1987;35(3):189–97.

86. Rudman D, Drinka PJ, Wilson CR, et al. Relations of endogenous anabolic hormones and physical activity to bone mineral density and lean body mass in elderly men. Clin Endocrinol 1994;40(5):653–61.

87. Fink H, Ewing SK, Ensrud KE, et al. Association of testosterone and estradiol deficiency with osteoporosis and rapid bone loss in older men. J Clin Endocrinol Metab 2006;91(10):3908–15.

88. Mellstrom D, Johnell O, Ljunggren O, et al. Free testosterone is an independent predictor of BMD and prevalent fractures in elderly men: MrOS Sweden. J Bone Miner Res 2006;21(4):529–35.

89. Ensrud K, Lewis CE, Lambert LC, et al. Osteoporotic Fractures in Men MrOS Study Research Group. Endogenous sex steroids, weight change and rates of hip bone loss in older men: the MrOS study. Osteoporos Int 2006;17(9):1329–36.

90. Nayak S, Liu H, Michaud K, et al. Cost-effectivess of alternative screening strategies for osteoporosis in postmenopausal women. 2006; Available at: http://smdm.confex.com. Accessed August 10, 2011.

91. Schousboe J, Ensrud KE, Nyman JA, et al. Universal bone densitometry, screening combined with alendronate therapy for those diagnosed with osteoporosis in highly cost-effective for elderly women. J Am Geriatr Soc 2005;53(10):1697–704.

92. Schousboe J, Taylor BC, Fink HA, et al. Cost-effectiveness of bone densitometry followed by treatment of osteoporosis in older men. JAMA 2007;298(6):629–37.

93. Bolland M, Grey AB, Gamble GD, et al. Effect of osteoporosis treatment on mortality: a meta-analysis. J Clin Endocrinol Metab 2010;95(3):1174–81.

94. National Osteoporosis Foundation. Clinician's Guide to Prevention and Treatment of Osteoporosis. 2008. Available at: http://www.nof.org/sites/default/files/pdfs/NOF_Clinicians_Guide2008.pdf, 2011. Accessed August 10, 2011.

95. Curtis J, Adachi JD, Saag KG. Bridging the osteoporosis quality chasm. J Bone Miner Res 2009;24:3–7.

96. Papaioannou A, Kennedy CC, Loannidis G, et al. The osteoporosis care gap in men with fragility fractures: the Canadian Multicenter Osteoporosis Study. Osteoporos Int 2008;19:581–7.

97. Kiebzak GM, Beinart GA, Perser K, et al. Undertreatment of osteoporosis in men with hip fracture. Arch Intern Med 2002;162(19):2217–22.

98. Force AHT. American Association of Clinical Endocrinologists medical guidelines for clinical practice for the evaluation and treatment of hypogonadism in adult male patients - 2002 update. 2002. Available at: http://www.touchgroupplc.com/pdf/790/2-aacehtf.pdf. Accessed August 10, 2011.

99. Arisaka O, Arisaka M, Nakayama Y, et al. Effect of testosterone on bone density and bone metabolism in adolescent male hypogonadism. Metabolism 1995;44:419–23.

100. van der Werff ten Bosch JJ, Bot A. Some skeletal dimensions of males with isolated gonadotrophin deficiency. Neth J Med 1992;41:259–63.

101. Adler RA, Hochberg MC. Glucocorticoid-induced osteoporosis in men. Endocrinol Invest 2011;34:481–4.

102. Grossman JM, Gordon R, Ranganath VK, et al. American College of Rheumatology 2010 recommendations for the prevention and treatment of glucocorticoid-induced osteoporosis. Arthritis Care Res (Hoboken) 2010;62(11):1515–26.

103. Reid IR, Wattie DJ, Evans MC, et al. Testosterone therapy in glucocorticoid-treated men. Arch Intern Med 1996;15:1173–7.

Update on Glucocorticoid-Induced Osteoporosis

Michael Maricic, MD[a,b,*]

KEYWORDS

- Glucocorticoids • Osteoporosis • Fractures
- Bisphosphonates • Teriparatide • Osteoblasts

Harvey Cushing first described the association between excess endogenous glucocorticoids and fractures in 1932.[1] Within a few years after the introduction of prednisone to treat rheumatoid arthritis by Philip Hench and colleagues,[2] the deleterious skeletal effects of exogenous glucocorticoids, including vertebral compression fractures, were reported.[3] Glucocorticoid-induced bone loss is the most common form of secondary osteoporosis, and fractures are glucocorticoids' most common adverse effect.[4] Glucocorticoids are used by 0.5% to 2.5% of adults, thus glucocorticoid-induced osteoporosis (GIOP) is one of the most common iatrogenic complications in clinical practice.[5] Whether the patient will develop osteoporosis and fractures depends not only on the daily and cumulative dose of glucocorticoids but also on several other concomitant factors, including the patient's baseline bone mineral density (BMD), age, sex, hormonal status, underlying disease for which the patient is being treated, and perhaps individual differences in sensitivity to glucocorticoids.

PATHOGENESIS OF GLUCOCORTICOID-INDUCED BONE LOSS

The most common histomorphometric finding in GIOP is a decrease in bone mass, most commonly seen in those parts of the skeleton with a high degree of cancellous bone, although cortical bone is not spared.[6] Glucocorticoids have both direct and indirect effects on bone, and affect both bone formation and resorption. Glucocorticoid-

Disclosure: The author has received research grant support and consultant fees from Merck, Proctor and Gamble, Eli Lilly, Novartis, and Amgen.
[a] Department of Medicine, University of Arizona School of Medicine, 1501 North Campbell, Tucson, AZ 85724, USA
[b] Catalina Pointe Rheumatology, 7520 North Oracle Road, Suite 100, Tucson, AZ 85704, USA
* University of Arizona School of Medicine, Tucson, AZ 85724.
E-mail address: mikemaricic@msn.com

induced osteoporosis occurs in two phases, a rapid phase of bone loss mediated through osteoclastic bone resorption and a later phase of bone loss caused by decreased bone formation.

Among the indirect effects, glucocorticoids cause a decrease in intestinal calcium absorption and an increase in the urinary excretion of calcium. Although secondary hyperparathyroidism had been thought to play a role in GIOP, elevated parathyroid hormone levels are not consistently found, and histomorphometric analysis of bone biopsies from patients with GIOP reveal decreased bone remodeling rather than the increased remodeling seen with secondary hyperparathyroidism.[6,7]

Another indirect effect of glucocorticoids on bone metabolism is through inhibition of gonadotropin secretion, leading to hypogonadism. Enhanced bone resorption ensues, at least in part, because of enhanced secretion of cytokines such as interleukin-6, tumor necrosis factor α, and macrophage-colony stimulating factor (M-CSF).[8]

A critical system involved in the coupling of bone formation and resorption is the RANK-L (receptor activator of nuclear factor-κB ligand)-RANK-OPG (osteoprotegerin) system. Under the influence of several cytokines and hormones such as tumor necrosis factor-α, parathyroid hormone, 1,25-dihydroxyvitamin D, and so forth., RANK-L is secreted by osteoblasts, then binds to and activates its receptor RANK on the surface of osteoclast precursors and induces osteoclastogenesis.[9] OPG is a natural inhibitor of RANK-L, preventing RANK-L from binding to its osteoclast receptor.

Glucocorticoids increase the expression of RANK-L and M-CSF,[10] and decrease OPG expression in osteoblasts and stromal cells. Glucocorticoids also increase the expression of interleukin-6, which stimulates osteoclastogenesis,[11] and downregulate the expression of interferon-β, an inhibitor of osteoclastogenesis.[12] These changes result in an initial increase in the number of osteoclasts capable of resorbing bone. Glucocorticoids initially also decrease the apoptosis of osteoclasts.[13] Eventually glucocorticoids deplete the population of osteoblasts as described below, which leads to decreased RANK-L and M-CSF expression by osteoblasts with a consequent decrease in osteoclast number.

The most significant mechanism of glucocorticoid-induced bone loss is decreased bone formation. Glucocorticoid exposure leads to a decrease in the number of osteoblasts, both by decreasing the formation of osteoblasts and by increasing osteoblast apoptosis.[14] Pluripotent bone marrow stromal cells have the ability to differentiate into several cells of the mesenchymal lineage, including either osteoblasts or adipocytes. Glucocorticoids shift the differentiation of pluripotent stromal cells away from osteoblasts toward the adipocyte lineage through regulation of nuclear factors of the CAAT enhancer-binding protein family and by induction of peroxisome proliferator activated receptor γ (PPARγ).[15,16] Glucocorticoids also suppress canonical Wnt-β-catenin signaling, a key regulator of osteoblastogenesis.[17] The bone morphogenetic protein (BMP) pathway, involved in stimulating osteoblast differentiation and bone formation, is also suppressed by glucocorticoids.[18]

In addition to their effects on osteoblastogenesis, glucocorticoids also have effects on bone matrix (inhibition of type I collagen synthesis and increased collagenase production)[19] and on skeletal growth factors (glucocorticoids downregulate transcription of the insulin growth factor I gene and its binding proteins).[20]

Osteocytes are thought to participate in the detection and healing of bone microdamage. Accelerated apoptosis of osteocytes could lead to accumulation of bone microdamage, and diminished bone quality and strength independent of BMD.[21] Increased osteocyte apoptosis has been documented in patients with GIOP.[14]

GLUCOCORTICOID EFFECTS ON BONE MINERAL DENSITY

Glucocorticoids affect both trabecular and cortical bone mass; however, bone loss is usually most marked in trabecular bone, due to its high surface area and high metabolic activity. Using quantitative computed tomography (QCT), a sensitive measure of trabecular bone density, declines of lumbar spine BMD of 8.2% within 20 weeks have been demonstrated.[22] After discontinuation of glucocorticoids, the lumbar spine BMD increased by 5.2%. Several studies have shown that bone loss is similar in men and women (both postmenopausal and premenopausal women). Fractures are more likely to occur in those with the lowest baseline bone mass, thus most studies demonstrate highest fracture rates in postmenopausal women.

GLUCOCORTICOID EFFECTS ON FRACTURE RISK

Glucocorticoid use increases the risk of both vertebral and nonvertebral fractures. In a study using an administrative claims database in the United States, Steinbuch and colleagues[23] compared fracture risk in glucocorticoid users to age-matched and sex-matched controls. The adjusted relative risk (RR) among users of glucocorticoids compared with controls was 2.92 for vertebral fractures, 1.68 for nonvertebral fractures, 1.87 for hip fractures, and 1.75 for any fracture.

Kanis and colleagues[24] studied the relationship between use of glucocorticoids and fracture risk in a meta-analysis of data from 7 cohort studies of 42,000 men and women. Both current and past use of glucocorticoids was an important predictor of fracture risk that was independent of prior fracture and BMD. No significant difference in risk was seen between men and women. For osteoporotic fracture, the range of RR was 1.71 to 2.63, and for hip fracture 2.38 to 4.42. Based on this and similar studies, *ever*-glucocorticoid use is incorporated as a major risk factor in the World Health Organization (WHO) Fracture Risk Assessment tool (FRAX) score.

The largest study examining the relationship between oral glucocorticoid use and fractures was the United Kingdom General Practice Database (GPDB) study reported by van Staa and colleagues.[25] This study compared the relative rates of fracture in 244,235 patients receiving oral glucocorticoids with age-matched and sex-matched controls. An average daily dose of prednisolone as low as 5 mg per day significantly increased the risk of spine and hip fracture. The most important risk for fracture in GIOP is the *daily* rather than the cumulative dose of oral glucocorticoids. The risk of nonvertebral fracture increases exponentially for daily doses of more than 20 mg prednisolone per day.[26] Fracture risk rises within 3 months of starting glucocorticoids, and falls after discontinuation within 1 year of stopping therapy. However, this increased risk does not fall completely back to baseline,[25] so that even prior users of glucocorticoids have an increased fracture risk irrespective of BMD.[24]

Several epidemiologic studies have reported an increased risk of fracture and lower BMD in patients using inhaled glucocorticoids.[27,28] Whether this is due to the glucocorticoids themselves or the underlying disease is controversial. A large cohort study performed by van Staa and colleagues[28] using the GPDB demonstrated that users of respiratory medications ($\beta2$ agonists) other than inhaled glucocorticoids are also associated with an increased risk of fracture, suggesting that the excess risk may be at least in part due to the underlying respiratory disease rather than to the inhaled glucocorticoids.

Other concomitant factors play a role in bone loss and fractures, including the underlying disease state for which glucocorticoids are given (eg, rheumatoid arthritis, lupus), individual differences in sensitivity to glucocorticoids, and the age and hormonal status of the patient. Although men and women are both susceptible to GIOP, the highest fracture rates are seen in postmenopausal women.

In a large cross-sectional, outpatient-based study of 551 postmenopausal women given glucocorticoids for different disease states, the prevalence of asymptomatic vertebral fractures was compared. The overall prevalence of asymptomatic vertebral fractures was greater than 37% and increased with age. Fourteen percent of patients had more than one symptomatic vertebral fracture. When controlled for age, glucocorticoid cumulative dose, duration of therapy, and personal history of fractures, the adjusted prevalence of vertebral fracture was 30.77% for systemic lupus erythematosus, 33.78% for rheumatoid arthritis, 37.78% for asthma/chronic obstructive pulmonary disease, 43.30% for polymyalgia rheumatica, and 43.36% for diseases grouped as other vasculidities/connective tissue diseases.[29]

BMD THRESHOLD FOR FRACTURES IN GLUCOCORTICOID-INDUCED OSTEOPOROSIS

The WHO criteria for the densitometric diagnosis of osteoporosis (T-score <-2.5) were developed based on the relationship of the prevalence of fractures in postmenopausal Caucasian females to the prevalence of T-scores below a certain level in the same population.[30] The same type of large epidemiologic study does not exist for glucocorticoid-treated patients.

To answer the question of whether fracture rates occur at a higher BMD or T-score in patients on glucocorticoids, Van Staa and colleagues[31] analyzed the relationship between BMD and vertebral fracture in postmenopausal women taking glucocorticoids. The investigators compared the incidence of fracture in the placebo groups from the risedronate prevention[32] and treatment[33] trials with the 1-year fracture risk of postmenopausal women not taking glucocorticoids in 3 other trials. In the BMD threshold analysis, even though the women taking glucocorticoids were younger (64.7 vs 74.1 years old), had less prevalent fractures (42.9% vs 58.3%), and had higher mean lumbar T-score (-1.8 vs -2.6) and femoral neck T-score (-1.9 vs -2.6) than the nonglucocorticoid users, the risk of fracture was higher in the glucocorticoid users than in the nonglucocorticoid users (adjusted RR 5.7 (95% confidence interval [CI] 2.57–12.54). Thus, fracture incidence was markedly higher in the glucocorticoid users at any given level of BMD.

NONPHARMACOLOGIC INTERVENTIONS

The 2010 American College of Rheumatology recommendations for the prevention and treatment of glucocorticoid-induced osteoporosis provide several suggestions for nonpharmacologic interventions.[34] The use and dose of systemic glucocorticoids should be minimized whenever possible. Fall risk assessment, smoking cessation, and alcohol cessation should be advised for all patients. Exercises to improve lower extremity strength and balance are particularly important in glucocorticoid-treated patients in whom glucocorticoid-induced myopathy may also lead to an increased risk of falls and fracture. Counseling on calcium and vitamin D intake is recommended for all patients receiving chronic glucocorticoids. Recommended calcium intake (supplements plus dietary intake) should be in the range of 1200 to 1500 mg per day. Vitamin D intake should be in the range of 800 to 1000 IU daily or whatever is necessary to achieve "therapeutic" levels of 25-OH vitamin D.

A 2-year trial of 65 rheumatoid arthritis patients treated chronically with low-dose prednisone (approximately 5 mg/d) randomized to placebo or daily 1000 mg of calcium carbonate and 500 IU of ergocalciferol demonstrated that those given the daily supplements demonstrated gains in BMD of 0.7% at lumbar spine and 0.9%

at the greater trochanter annually compared with losses of −2.0% and −0.9% at these sites in the placebo group.[35] A meta-analysis on the effectiveness of treatments for GIOP concluded that calcium plus vitamin D was more effective than no treatment or calcium alone at the lumbar spine.[36] A meta-analysis of active vitamin D3 analogues in GIOP found that they preserve bone density more effectively than no treatment, plain vitamin D3, and/or calcium.[37] However, bisphosphonates were found to be more effective in preserving bone and decreasing the risk of vertebral fractures than active vitamin D3 analogues.

Calcium and vitamin D should be considered necessary but not sufficient for patients receiving chronic glucocorticoids, as they do not reduce fracture risk to the same degree as bisphosphonates and/or teriparatide.

BISPHOSPHONATES

Bisphosphonates were the first class of agents demonstrated to be effective for the prevention and treatment of GIOP. Most trials have examined their efficacy on BMD as the primary end point; however, post hoc analyses also support an effect on fracture reduction (mainly in the group at highest risk, namely postmenopausal women). In the United States, risedronate (5 mg/d) is approved by the Food and Drug Administration (FDA) for the prevention and/or treatment of GIOP, and alendronate (5 mg/d for males and premenopausal females, and 10 mg/d for postmenopausal females not receiving estrogen therapy) is approved for the treatment of GIOP. Although commonly used in clinical practice, neither weekly alendronate nor weekly or monthly risedronate have been FDA-approved for GIOP.

In studies of patients receiving glucocorticoids, daily alendronate, daily risedronate, and cyclic etidronate (400 mg/d for 2 weeks followed by a 10-week rest period) have demonstrated significant increases in BMD at both the hip and spine, and post hoc analyses have demonstrated reductions in vertebral fracture risk (all compared with calcium and vitamin D alone). In the alendronate GIOP trial reported by Saag and colleagues,[38] there were too few patients with new vertebral fractures after 1 year, so that fracture reduction was not significant. After 2 years, a significant reduction of 89% in vertebral fractures was demonstrated.[39] A pooling of the risedronate prevention and treatment studies demonstrated a significant 70% reduction in vertebral fractures after 1 year compared with calcium and vitamin D alone.[40] Cyclic etidronate was demonstrated to reduce the risk of new vertebral fractures by 85% over 1 year compared with placebo.[41] These studies were not head to head, and thus no inferences on superiority of fracture reduction should be drawn from these numbers.

A meta-regression analysis[42] comparing the efficacy of therapies used for the treatment of glucocorticoid-induced osteoporosis determined that bisphosphonates were the most effective class of drugs to preserve vertebral BMD, with an effect size of 1.03 (95% CI 0.85–1.17) compared with vitamin D (0.46; 95% CI 0.27–0.62), or calcitonin (0.51; 95% CI 0.33–0.67) therapy. When combined with vitamin D, the effect size of bisphosphonates further increased to 1.31 (95% CI 1.07–1.50).

In patients who cannot tolerate oral bisphosphonates, intravenous zoledronic acid and subcutaneous teriparatide are now available. Prior to the advent of intravenous zoledronic acid, intravenous pamidronate was found to be a useful agent in some studies.[43] Pamidronate is rarely used any longer for GIOP. Not only is the infusion time longer (2–3 hours for pamidronate vs 15–30 minutes for zoledronic acid), but pamidronate is given every 3 months versus once yearly. If pamidronate were to be given, the same restriction on patients with a creatinine clearance of less than 35 mL/min must be observed.

Ibandronate is approved for monthly oral use in the treatment of postmenopausal osteoporosis but not in GIOP. However, there has been a study suggesting potential efficacy of intravenous ibandronate in GIOP. One hundred and fifteen patients receiving long-term glucocorticoids (average daily dose 10 mg prednisone) were randomized to receive either 500 mg of calcium and 1 μg of alfacalcidiol daily, or calcium plus infusions of 2 mg intravenous ibandronate every 3 months.[44] At 3 years, BMD was increased 13.3% at the lumbar spine and 5.2% at the femoral neck in the ibandronate group compared with the alfacalcidiol group (2.6% and 1.9%, respectively). Although not specifically powered to detect a reduction in fracture risk, the incidence of new vertebral fractures in the ibandronate group (8.6%) compared with the alfacalcidiol group (22.8%) was a 62% RR reduction ($P = .043$). Intravenous ibandronate is not currently approved for GIOP, and should not be administered to patients with a creatinine clearance of less than 35 mL/min because of the potential for renal toxicity.

Intravenous zoledronic acid has now been demonstrated to be effective in the prevention and treatment of GIOP and is approved in the United States for this indication at the dose of 5 mg once yearly. Zoledronic acid is a third-generation bisphosphonate, which has 2 nitrogen atoms contained in a heterocyclic imidazole ring. Zoledronic acid has been shown to be the most potent inhibitor of farnesyl diphosphate synthase (the main mechanism by which nitrogen-containing bisphosphonates exert their cellular effects) to date.[45] Because it is administered as a once-yearly infusion, zoledronic acid has the potential to ensure adherence and avoid upper gastrointestinal irritation associated with oral bisphosphonates.

The safety and efficacy of 5 mg intravenous zoledronic acid for treatment and prevention of GIOP was assessed in HORIZON-GIOP, a 1-year randomized, double-blind, active controlled study of 833 men and women treated with 7.5 mg/d or more oral prednisone (or equivalent) who were expected to remain on treatment for at least 12 months.[46] Patients were stratified into the prevention and treatment groups according to the duration of glucocorticoid use at study entry (≤3 months and >3 months, respectively). Patients received a single 5-mg zoledronic acid infusion or 5 mg oral risedronate per day for 12 months. All patients received 1000 mg calcium plus 400 to 1000 IU vitamin D. The primary end point was percentage change from baseline in lumbar spine BMD. Zoledronic acid produced significantly greater increases in lumbar spine BMD than risedronate in both the treatment and prevention subpopulations at 12 months (treatment subpopulation: zoledronic acid 4.1% vs risedronate 2.7%; $P = .0001$; prevention subpopulation: zoledronic acid 2.6% vs risedronate 0.6%; $P<.0001$).

In the HORIZON-GIOP trials, adverse events occurred more frequently in the intravenous zoledronic acid treatment group than in the risedronate group during the first 3 days after infusion; these were mainly transient postdose flulike symptoms. The overall incidence of adverse events was otherwise similar. Intravenous zoledronic acid should not be given to patients with significant renal impairment (creatinine clearance <35 mL/min), due to the potential for worsening renal function and acute renal failure in those patients.

TERIPARATIDE (PARATHYROID HORMONE)

Teriparatide is now approved for the treatment of glucocorticoid-induced osteoporosis, and its anabolic activity in stimulating and prolonging the life span of osteoblasts suggests an important role in GIOP. Teriparatide induces differentiation of bone lining cells and preosteoblasts into osteoblasts, stimulates the activity of existing osteoblasts to form new bone, and decreases apoptosis of both osteoblasts and osteocytes.[47]

A 12-month trial of females with low bone mass (T-score ≤−2.5) who were on long-term estrogen and glucocorticoids (mean 8.5 mg of prednisone daily for an average of 13 years) was performed to compare the additive effects of subcutaneous daily human parathyroid hormone (PTH(1–84)) with placebo.[48] Both groups received 1500 mg calcium and 800 IU vitamin D per day. BMD at the lumbar spine was significantly greater in the combination PTH and estrogen group (11% increase by dual-energy x-ray absorptiometry (DXA) and 33% by QCT scanning) compared with the estrogen-alone group at 12 months). Increases in femoral neck BMD were significant in the combination group at 24 months. The effect on BMD was sustained for 1 year following the discontinuation of PTH(1–84) and the continuation of estrogen.[49]

In an 18-month active controlled, double-blind clinical trial of women and men with GIOP,[50] subjects taking at least 5 mg/d prednisone equivalent for 3 or more months were randomized to receive either daily teriparatide (TPTD), 20 μg/d (n = 214) or alendronate (ALN), 10 mg/d (n = 214). The primary objective of the study was the change in lumbar spine BMD measured by DXA at 18 months. Secondary outcomes were change in BMD at the total hip, change in biochemical markers of bone turnover, vertebral fractures, and safety. Vertebral fractures were assessed at a central coordinating center. At baseline, for ALN versus TPTD, respectively, the median glucocorticoid dose was 7.8 versus 7.5 mg/d, spine T-scores were (mean ± SE) −2.5 ± 0.1 versus −2.4 ± 0.1, and 25% versus 30% of patients had a prevalent vertebral fracture.

The mean (±SE) percent changes in lumbar spine BMD were greater with TPTD (7.2% ± 0.7%) than with ALN (3.4% ± 0.7%) ($P<.001$). At 12 months, bone mineral density at the total hip increased more with TPTD than with ALN. Fewer new vertebral fractures occurred in more patients in the ALN (n = 10; 6.1%) than in the TPTD group (n = 1; 0.6%) ($P = .004$), with no significant difference in the number of patients with new nonvertebral fractures (ALN n = 8 [3.7%] vs TPTD n = 12 [5.6%], $P = .493$).

An analysis to examine the effect of gender and menopausal status on changes in BMD, change in biochemical markers of bone turnover, fracture incidence, and safety in subgroups of postmenopausal women, premenopausal women, and men with GIOP treated with teriparatide or alendronate in the aforementioned trial has been published.[51] At 18 months, increases in lumbar spine BMD were significantly greater in the TPTD group than in the ALN group in postmenopausal women (7.8% vs 3.7%, $P<.001$), premenopausal women (7.0% vs 0.7%, $P<.001$), and men (7.3% vs 3.7%, $P = .03$). A significant difference in hip BMD was found only in premenopausal women (TPTD 4.8 ± 1.3 vs ALN 1.8 ± 1.5, $P = .006$). More new vertebral fractures occurred in the ALN group than in the TPTD group in men (n = 4 [2.4%] vs n = 0, $P = .113$) and postmenopausal women (n = 6 [3.6%] vs n = 1 [0.6%], $P = .120$); no fractures occurred in premenopausal women.

The 36-month extension of this original 18-month trial demonstrated continued superiority of TPTD over ALN.[52] At 36 months, increases in BMD at the lumbar spine from baseline were 11.0% for TPTD versus 5.3% for ALN, at the total hip were 5.2% for TPTD versus 2.7% for ALN, and at the femoral neck were 6.3% for TPTD versus 2.4% for ALN. Fewer subjects had new vertebral fractures in the TPTD group (3 of 173 [1.7%]) than in the ALN group (13 of 169 [7.7%]).

Contraindications to the use of TPTD include children or young adults with open epiphyses, pregnant females, and patients with hyperparathyroidism, Paget disease of bone, osteomalacia, end-stage renal disease, primary or metastatic bone cancer, active nephrolithiasis or unexplained elevation of serum calcium, or alkaline phosphatase prior to initiation of therapy. Radiation therapy involving the skeleton excludes a patient from treatment with TPTD.

OTHER THERAPIES

Other pharmacologic options for the prevention of bone loss include nasal spray calcitonin, and hormone therapy or selective estrogen receptor modulators in women and testosterone in men. Studies of calcitonin in GIOP are limited, with conflicting data on its ability to prevent bone loss[53] and no studies that demonstrate fracture risk reduction. No studies currently exist examining the role of selective estrogen receptor modulators in GIOP. A few small studies of hormone therapy in GIOP have been performed. In one trial of postmenopausal women receiving prednisone for rheumatoid arthritis, those randomized to hormone therapy had a significant (3.4%) increase in their lumbar spine BMD compared with controls. There was no significant change in femoral neck BMD in either group.[54] Similar small studies of testosterone replacement in GIOP have been performed,[55] demonstrating increases in BMD at 1 year of 5% in hypogonadal asthmatic men treated with testosterone compared with controls. Increases in lean body mass (reflecting muscle mass) were also demonstrated in the testosterone-treated men.

Due to the increased risks of breast cancer and cardiovascular disease associated with long-term hormone therapy,[56] recommendations for its use as a primary treatment for GIOP cannot be made. Similar arguments could be made for testosterone replacement, for which the long-term adverse effects are unknown.[57] These therapies are most likely to be appropriate in the patient on glucocorticoids for whom deficiencies of these hormones lead to vasomotor symptoms, loss of libido, and so forth, and whereby specific replacement could enhance the patient's quality of life for reasons other than osteoporosis. In the 2010 American College of Rheumatology (ACR) recommendations for the prevention and treatment of GIOP, previously included hormone therapy and testosterone are no longer endorsed.

2010 AMERICAN COLLEGE OF RHEUMATOLOGY RECOMMENDATIONS FOR THE PREVENTION AND TREATMENT OF GIOP

In 2010, the ACR updated their recommendations for the prevention and treatment of glucocorticoid-induced osteoporosis.[34] The rationale for updating and reappraising the previous 2001 ACR guidelines include:

1. Guideline development methodology has evolved from a more informal consensus approach to a more rigorous process
2. Additional therapies (zoledronic acid and teriparatide) and new data on therapies included in the previous recommendations have become available
3. Updated approaches to identify patients at highest risk for fracture have been developed (the WHO FRAX and 2008 revised National Osteoporosis Foundation guidelines for the treatment of prevention of osteoporosis).

The recommendations of the ACR committee were based on a rigorous systematic review of research articles published between 1966 and August 20, 2008, and the work of a primary Core Executive Panel (CEP). The CEP used the Research and Development/University of California at Los Angeles (RAND/UCLA) appropriateness method with the assistance of two expert panels: the Expert Advisory Panel which framed the development of recommendations, and the task force panel which voted on the specific recommendations. Full details of that process can be found in the publication of these recommendations.[34] The current recommendations do not address inhaled glucocorticoids, pulse intravenous glucocorticoids, or GIOP in transplant recipients.

The previous 2001 ACR recommendations included counseling of patients receiving glucocorticoid therapy on smoking cessation or avoidance or limiting excessive alcohol intake, weight-bearing activities, calcium and vitamin D intake and supplementation, and obtaining baseline and follow-up BMD measurement. Recommendations for counseling and monitoring are now expanded to include fall risk assessment, height measurement, 25-hydroxyvitamin D measurement, and consideration of evaluation for prevalent and incident fragility fractures by vertebral fracture assessment (by DXA) or radiographic imaging of the spine. Calcium and vitamin D supplementation is now recommended for any duration of glucocorticoid use.

Recommendations for pharmacologic intervention are now guided by the patient's overall clinical risk instead of T-scores alone. Because factors other than T-scores such as age, weight, current smoking, and so forth contribute to fracture risk, the ACR recommendations are guided in part by the FRAX score of patient's overall clinical risk profile.

Using the FRAX calculator, the expert advisory panel defined a 10-year risk of major osteoporotic fracture of 10% or less as low risk, 10% to 20% as medium risk, and greater than 20% or a T-score of less than or equal to −2.5 or a history of fragility fracture as high risk.

Fracture risk assessment may be increased or "shifted to a higher category" in patients who have additional risk factors not considered in FRAX alone. Because FRAX uses an average glucocorticoid dose to calculate a 10-year probability of a major osteoporotic fracture, those receiving higher daily or cumulative dose of oral glucocorticoids, and intravenous pulse glucocorticoids, may have an increased risk of fracture. A declining central BMD measurement that exceeds a least significant change on therapy may be another reason that clinicians would move the patient to higher risk category. All of these factors need to be considered in the assessment of the patient, and may shift an individual into a greater category risk than that derived using FRAX alone.

The basic approach to postmenopausal women and men older than 50 years who are initiating or receiving glucocorticoid therapy is to provide universal counseling and assessment of risk factors. The prescribing provider should then determine the patient risk category using the FRAX score or tables provided by the ACR (**Fig. 1**) to stratify the patient into low, medium, or high risk. Recommendations on which pharmacologic agents could be used are given depending on whether the patient is considered to be low, medium, or high risk (**Fig. 2**). It must be recognized that these recommendations are based on the consensus opinion and voting of the expert panels, and not on comparative data or head-to-head trials of these pharmacologic agents in these specific risk groups. No matter which therapy is chosen, patients should then be monitored with assessment of osteoporosis medication compliance, annual height measurement, and serial BMD testing. Consideration of annual serum 25-hydroxyvitamin D measurement and assessment of incident fragility fractures is also recommended.

Recommendations are also given for premenopausal women and men younger than 50 with a history of fragility fractures (**Fig. 3**). The recommendations for premenopausal women and younger men are constrained by the paucity of evidence for fracture risk in the treatment of GIOP in these populations.

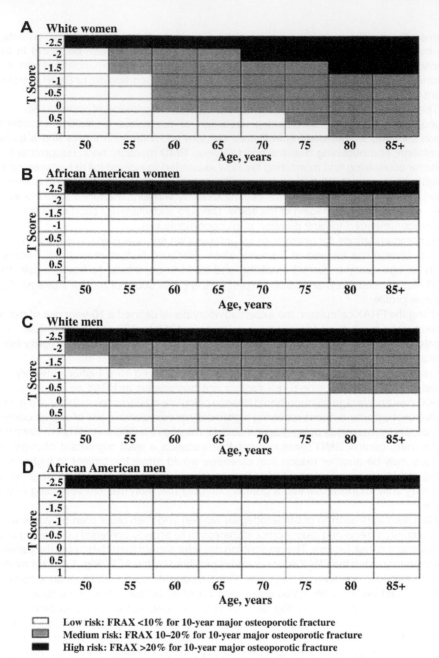

Fig. 1. Typical examples of postmenopausal women and men older than 50 years with a history of glucocorticoid use at high, medium, and low risk of fracture in the absence of other risk factors in (*A*) white women, (*B*) African American women, (*C*) white men, and (*D*) African American men. High-, medium-, and low-risk patient classification is based on an approximation of FRAX 3.0 using age, sex, race, T-score, and the presence of glucocorticoids for the calculation, with all other risk factors in the FRAX calculation absent. (*From* Grossman JM, Gordon R, Ranganath VK, et al. Recommendations for the prevention and treatment of glucocorticoid-induced osteoporosis. Arthritis Care Res 2010;62:1517; with permission.)

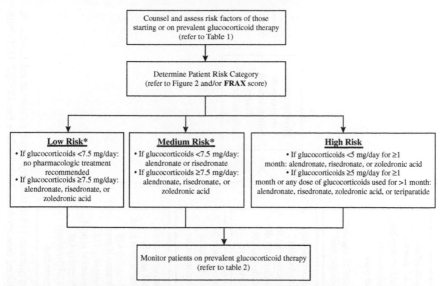

Fig. 2. Approach to postmenopausal women and men older than 50 years initiating or receiving glucocorticoid therapy. * For low- and medium-risk patients, recommendations are for an anticipated or prevalent duration of 3 months or more of glucocorticoid treatment. (*From* Grossman JM, Gordon R, Ranganath VK, et al. Recommendations for the prevention and treatment of glucocorticoid-induced osteoporosis. Arthritis Care Res 2010;62:1519; with permission.)

Limitations of the 2010 ACR recommendations include the limited quality of available evidence and the limitations of the FRAX tool around which the categorization of high, medium, and low risk for fracture assessment of patients is based. The FRAX calculator uses only bone density at the hip. Patients with glucocorticoid-induced osteoporosis frequently lose bone mass first in trabecular bone (the spine), which may lead to an underestimation of vertebral fracture risk. Also, many of the clinical risk factors in FRAX are dichotomous (yes/no) and do not take into account dose response (ie, dose of glucocorticoids, number of cigarettes smoked, number of alcoholic drinks, number of previous fractures). FRAX provides hazard ratios based on an average dose or exposure for these variables.[58] Because fracture risk associated with glucocorticoid use is clearly dose related, this limits the use of the FRAX tool in this instance.

Kanis and colleagues[59] have recently published an article giving guidance for the adjustment of FRAX according to the dose of glucocorticoids. Dose responses for fracture risk during exposure to glucocorticoids were derived from the GPDB[25,26] and were used to adjust the RRs for glucocorticoid use in FRAX. For "all ages," the probability of a major osteoporotic fracture is decreased by about 20% for low-dose exposure (<2.5 mg daily of prednisolone or equivalent) and increased by about 15% for high-dose exposure (>7.5 mg daily). For all ages, the probability of hip fractures is decreased by about 35% for low-dose exposure and increased by about 20% for high doses. For patients on medium doses (2.5–7.5 mg daily), the unadjusted FRAX values for hip and major osteoporotic fractures can be used. The adjustments vary somewhat depending the on age of the patient, as shown in **Table 1**.

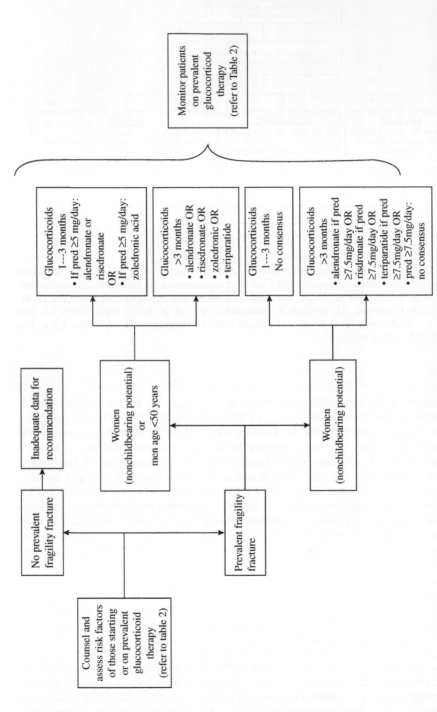

Fig. 3. Approach to premenopausal women and men younger than 50 years starting or receiving glucocorticoid therapy. (*From* Grossman JM, Gordon R, Ranganath VK, et al. Recommendations for the prevention and treatment of glucocorticoid-induced osteoporosis. Arthritis Care Res 2010;62:1520; with permission.)

Table 1
Percentage adjustment of 10-year probabilities of a hip fracture or a major osteoporotic fracture by age according to dose of glucocorticoids

Dose	Prednisolone Equivalent (mg/d)	Age (y)						All Ages
		40	50	60	70	80	90	
Hip Fracture								
Low	<2.5	−40	−40	−40	−40	−30	−30	−35
Medium[a]	2.5–7.5	—	—	—	—	—	—	—
High	≥7.5	+25	+25	+25	+20	+10	+10	+20
Major Osteoporotic Fracture								
Low	<2.5	−20	−20	−15	−20	−20	−20	−20
Medium[a]	2.5–7.5	—	—	—	—	—	—	—
High	≥7.5	+20	+20	+15	+15	+10	+10	+15

[a] No adjustment.
Data from Kanis JA, Johansson H, Oden A, et al. Guidance for adjustment of FRAX according to the dose of glucocorticoids. Osteoporos Int 2011;22:813.

SUMMARY

Despite the knowledge of the fracture risk associated with glucocorticoids, published guidelines, and the availability of effective prophylaxis and treatment, measurement of bone density and institution of medications to prevent bone loss in GIOP is suboptimal,[60,61] including among specialty physicians.[62] Systematic health care GIOP programs[63] and evidence-based intervention programs[64] for the cost-effective management of GIOP are being developed, which may improve patient management. Continued education, dissemination of guidelines, and other innovative approaches will be necessary to make a more substantial impact on this disorder.

REFERENCES

1. Cushing H. The basophil adenomas of the pituitary body and their clinical manifestations (pituitary basophilism). Bull Johns Hopkins Hosp 1932;50:137–95.
2. Hench PH, Kendall P, Slocumb CH, et al. The effect of a hormone of the adrenal cortex (17-hydroxy-11-dehydrocorticosterone; compound E) and of pituitary adrenocorticotropic hormone on rheumatoid arthritis. Mayo Clin Proc 1949; 24(8):181–97.
3. Curtis PH, Clark WS, Herndon CH. Vertebral fractures resulting from prolonged cortisone and corticotropin therapy. JAMA 1954;156:467–9.
4. Saag KG, Koehnke R, Caldwell JR, et al. Low dose long-term corticosteroid therapy in rheumatoid arthritis: an analysis of serious adverse events. Am J Med 1994;96(2):115–23.
5. van Staa TP, Cooper C, Abenhaim L, et al. Utilization of oral corticosteroids in the United Kingdom. Q J Med 2000;93:105–11.
6. Dempster DW. Bone histomorphometry in glucocorticoid-induced osteoporosis. J Bone Miner Res 1989;4:137–41.
7. Carbonare LD, Bertoldo F, Valenti MT, et al. Histomorphometric analysis of glucocorticoid-induced osteoporosis. Micron 2005;36:645–52.
8. Weitzmann MN, Pacifici R. Estrogen deficiency and bone loss: an inflammatory tale. J Clin Invest 2006;116:1186–94.

9. Hofbauer LC, Gori F, Riggs BL, et al. Stimulation of osteoprotegerin ligand and inhibition of osteoprotegerin production by glucocorticoids in human osteoblastic lineage cells: potential paracrine mechanisms of glucocorticoid-induced osteoporosis. Endocrinology 1999;140:4382–9.

10. Alesci S, De Martino MU, Illias I. Glucocorticoid-induced osteoporosis: from basic mechanisms to clinical aspects. Neuroimmunomodulation 2005;12:1–19.

11. Dovio A, Perazzolo L, Saba L, et al. High-dose glucocorticoids increase serum levels of soluble II-6 receptor alpha and its ratio to soluble gp130: an additional mechanism for early increased bone resorption. Eur J Endocrinol 2006;154:745–51.

12. Takuma A, Kaneda T, Sato T, et al. Dexamethasone enhances osteoclasts formation synergistically with transforming growth factor-beta by stimulating the priming of osteoclast progenitors for differentiation into osteoclasts. J Biol Chem 2003;278:44667–74.

13. Jia D, O'Brien CA, Stewart SA, et al. Glucocorticoids act directly on osteoclasts to increase their life span and reduce bone density. Endocrinology 2006;147: 5592–9.

14. Weinstein RS, Jilka RL, Parfitt AM, et al. Inhibition of osteoblastogenesis and promotion of apoptosis of osteoblasts and osteocytes by glucocorticoids: potential mechanisms of their deleterious effects on bone. J Clin Invest 1998;102: 274–82, 25.

15. Canalis E. Glucocorticoid-induced osteoporosis: pathophysiology. In: Maricic M, Gluck O, editors. Bone disease in rheumatology. New York: Lippincott; 2005. p. 105–10.

16. Pereira RC, Delany AM, Canalis E. Effects of cortisol and bone morphogenetic protein-2 on stromal cell differentiation: correlation with CCAAT-enhancer binding protein expression. Bone 2002;30:685–91.

17. Ohnaka K, Tanabe M, Kawate H, et al. Glucocorticoid suppresses the canonical Wnt signal in human osteoblast. Biochem Biophys Res Commun 2005;329: 177–81.

18. Leclerc N, Lupen CA, Ho VV. Gene expression profiling of glucocorticoid-inhibited osteoblasts. J Mol Endocrinol 2004;33(1):175–93.

19. Delany AM, Jeffrey JJ, Rydziel S, et al. Cortisol increases interstitial collagenase expression in osteoblasts by post-transcriptional mechanisms. J Biol Chem 1995; 270:26607–12.

20. Delany AM, Durant D, Canalis E. Glucocorticoid suppression of IGF I transcription in osteoblasts. Mol Endocrinol 2001;15:1781–9.

21. Weinstein RS, Powers CC, Parfitt AM, et al. Preservation of osteocyte viability by bisphosphonates contributes to bone strength in glucocorticoid-treated mice independently of BMD: an unappreciated determinant of bone strength. J Bone Miner Res 2002;17(Suppl 1):S156.

22. Laan RF, van Riel PL, van de Putte LB, et al. Low-dose prednisone induces rapid reversible axial bone loss in patients with rheumatoid arthritis. Ann Intern Med 1993;119(10):963–8.

23. Steinbuch M, Thomas E, Youket E, et al. Oral glucocorticoid use is associated with an increased risk of fracture. Osteoporos Int 2004;15:323–8.

24. Kanis JA, Johannson H, Oden A, et al. A meta-analysis of prior corticosteroid use and fracture risk. J Bone Miner Res 2004;19:893–9.

25. van Staa T, Leufkens H, Abenhaim L, et al. Use of oral corticosteroids and risk of fractures. J Bone Miner Res 2000;15(6):993–1000.

26. van Staa TP, Leufkens HM, Abenhaim L, et al. Oral corticosteroids and fracture risk: relationship to daily and cumulative doses. Rheumatology 2000;39:1383–9.

27. Hubbard RB, Smith CJ, Smeeth L, et al. Inhaled corticosteroids and hip fracture: a population-based case-control study. Am J Respir Crit Care Med 2002;166: 1563–6.
28. van Staa TP, Leufkens HG, Cooper C. Use of inhaled corticosteroids and risk of fractures. J Bone Miner Res 2001;3:581–8.
29. Angeli A, Gugliemi G, Dovio A, et al. High prevalence of asymptomatic vertebral fractures in post-menopausal women receiving chronic glucocorticoid therapy; a cross-sectional outpatient study. Bone 2006;39:253–9.
30. World Health Organization. Assessment of fracture risk and its application to screening for postmenopausal osteoporosis. Technical report series 843. Geneva (Switzerland): WHO; 1994.
31. Van Staa TP, Laan RF, Barton IP, et al. Bone density threshold and other predictors of vertebral fracture in patients receiving oral glucocorticoid therapy. Arthritis Rheum 2003;48(11):3224–9.
32. Cohen S, Levy RM, Keller M, et al. Risedronate therapy prevents corticosteroid-induced bone loss: a twelve-month, multicenter, randomized, double-blind, placebo-controlled, parallel-group study. Arthritis Rheum 1999; 42(11):2309–18.
33. Reid DM, Hughes R, Laan RF. Efficacy and safety of daily risedronate in the treatment of corticosteroid-induced osteoporosis in men and women: a randomized trial. J Bone Miner Res 2000;15:1006–13.
34. Grossman JM, Gordon R, Ranganath VK, et al. Recommendations for the prevention and treatment of glucocorticoid-induced osteoporosis. Arthritis Care Res 2010;62:1515–26.
35. Buckley LM, Leib ES, Cartularo KS, et al. Calcium and vitamin D3 supplementation prevents bone loss in the spine secondary to low-dose corticosteroids in patients with rheumatoid arthritis. Ann Intern Med 1996;125:961–8.
36. Amin S, LaValley MP, Simms RW, et al. The role of vitamin D in corticosteroid-induced osteoporosis: a meta-analytic approach. Arthritis Rheum 1999;42: 1740–51.
37. de Nijs RN, Jacobs JW, Algra A, et al. Prevention and treatment of glucocorticoid-induced osteoporosis with active vitamin D3 analogues: a review with meta-analysis of randomized controlled trials including organ transplantation studies. Osteoporos Int 2004;15:589–602.
38. Saag KG, Emkey R, Schnitzer T, et al. Alendronate for the treatment and prevention glucocorticoid-induced osteoporosis. N Engl J Med 1998;339:292–9.
39. Adachi JD, Saag K, Emkey R, et al. Effects of alendronate for two years on BMD and fractures in patients receiving glucocorticoids. Arthritis Rheum 2001;44: 202–11.
40. Wallach S, Cohen S, Reid DM, et al. Effects of risedronate treatment on bone density an vertebral fracture in patients on corticosteroid therapy. Calcif Tissue Int 2000;67:277–85.
41. Adachi JD, Bensen WG, Brown J, et al. Intermittent etidronate therapy to prevent corticosteroid induced osteoporosis. N Engl J Med 1997;337:382–7.
42. Amin S, LaValley MP, Simms RW, et al. The comparative efficacy of drug therapies used for the management of corticosteroid-induced osteoporosis: a meta-regression. J Bone Miner Res 2002;17:1512–26.
43. Boutsen Y, Jamart J, Esselinckx W, et al. Primary prevention of glucocorticoid-induced osteoporosis with intravenous pamidronate and calcium: a prospective controlled 1-year study comparing a single infusion, an infusion given once every 3 months, and calcium alone. J Bone Miner Res 2001;16(1):104–12.

44. Ringe JD, Dorst A, Faber H, et al. Intermittent intravenous ibandronate injections reduce vertebral fracture risk in corticosteroid-induced osteoporosis: results from a long-term comparative study. Osteoporos Int 2003;14(10):801–7.

45. Green JR, Rogers MJ. Pharmacological profile of zoledronic acid: a highly potent inhibitor of bone resorption. Drug Dev Res 2002;55:210–24.

46. Reid DM, Devogelaer JP, Saag K, et al. Zoledronic acid and risedronate in the prevention and treatment of glucocorticoid-induced osteoporosis (HORIZON): a multicentre, double-blind, double-dummy randomised controlled trial. Lancet 2009;373:1253–63.

47. Canalis E, Giustina A, Bilizekian JP. Mechanisms of anabolic therapies for osteoporosis. N Engl J Med 2007;357:905–16.

48. Lane NE, Sanchez S, Modin GW, et al. Parathyroid hormone treatment can reverse corticosteroid-induced osteoporosis. Results of a randomized controlled clinical trial. J Clin Invest 1998;102(8):1627–33.

49. Lane NE, Sanchez S, Modin GW, et al. Bone mass continues to increase at the hip after parathyroid hormone treatment is discontinued in glucocorticoid induced osteoporosis: results of a randomized controlled clinical trial. J Bone Miner Res 2000;15(5):944–51.

50. Saag KG, Shane ES, Boonen S, et al. Teriparatide or alendronate in glucocorticoid-induced osteoporosis. N Engl J Med 2007;357:2028–39.

51. Langdahl BL, Marin F, Shane E, et al. Teriparatide versus alendronate for treating glucocorticoid-induced osteoporosis: analysis by gender and menopausal status. Osteoporos Int 2009;20:2095–103.

52. Saag KG, Zancetta JR, Devogelear JP, et al. Effects of teriparatide versus alendronate for treating glucocorticoid-induced osteoporosis: thirty six-month results of a randomized, double-blind controlled trial. Arthritis Rheum 2009; 60:3346–55.

53. Healey JH, Paget SA, Williams-Russo P, et al. A randomized controlled trial of salmon calcitonin to prevent bone loss in corticosteroid-treated temporal arteritis and polymyalgia rheumatica. Calcif Tissue Int 1996;58:73–80.

54. Hall GM, Daniels M, Doyle DV, et al. Effect of hormone replacement therapy on bone mass in rheumatoid arthritis patients treated with and without steroids. Arthritis Rheum 1994;37:1499–505.

55. Reid IR, Wattie DJ, Evans MC, et al. Testosterone therapy in glucocorticoid-treated men. Arch Intern Med 1996;156:1173–7.

56. Rossouw JW, Anderson GL, Prentice RL, et al. Risks and benefits of estrogen plus progestin in healthy post-menopausal women: principal results from the women's health initiative randomized controlled trial. JAMA 2002;288:321–33.

57. Rhoden EL, Morgentaler A. Risks of testosterone-replacement therapy and recommendations for monitoring. N Engl J Med 2004;350:482–92.

58. Kanis JA, Johnell O, Oden A, et al. FRAX and the assessment of fracture probability in men and women from the UK. Osteoporos Int 2008;18:1033–46.

59. Kanis JA, Johansson H, Oden A, et al. Guidance for adjustment of FRAX according to the dose of glucocorticoids. Osteoporos Int 2011;22:809–16.

60. Curtis JR, Westfall AO, Allison JJ, et al. Longitudinal patterns in the prevention of osteoporosis in Glucocorticoid-treated patients. Arthritis Rheum 2005;52: 2485–94.

61. Guzman-Clark JR, Fang MA, Fehl ME, et al. Barriers in the management of glucocorticoid-induced osteoporosis. Arthritis Rheum 2007;57:140–6.

62. Solomon DH, Katz JN, Jacobs JP, et al. Management of glucocorticoid-induced osteoporosis in patients with rheumatoid arthritis: rates and predictors of care in an academic rheumatology practice. Arthritis Rheum 2002;46:3136–42.
63. Newman ED, Matsko CK, Oleginski TP, et al. Glucocorticoid-induced osteoporosis program (GIOP): a normal, comprehensive and successful program with improved outcomes at one year. Osteoporos Int 2006;17:1428–34.
64. Beukelman T, Saag KG, Curtis JR. Cost-effectiveness of multifaceted implementation programs for the prevention of glucocorticoid-induced osteoporosis. Osteoporos Int 2010;21:1573–84.

The RANKL Pathway and Denosumab

Robin K. Dore, MD*

KEYWORDS

• Denosumab • RANKL • RANK • FREEDOM • Osteoporosis

Bone remodeling is a lifelong process in which old bone is replaced by new bone. This remodeling occurs in response to mechanical stresses and hormonal changes. This coordinated process of bone resorption and formation renews the skeleton while maintaining its structure. Bone remodeling also helps maintain mineral homeostasis, releasing calcium and phosphorus into the circulation. Bone remodeling occurs within discrete units called basic multicellular units or bone remodeling units (BMUs). These remodeling sites are found on both cortical and trabecular bone surfaces. The remodeling process results in the formation of a new osteon via a coordinated and sequential effort between osteoclasts and osteoblasts. Osteoclasts are tissue-specific macrophages created by the differentiation of monocyte/macrophage precursor cells at or near the bone surface. Their transformation from monocyte/macrophage lineage precursor cells into multinucleated cells is choreographed by a sequence of events that includes proliferation, differentiation, fusion, and activation.[1] Interleukins (IL-1, IL-4, IL-7, IL-11, IL-17), tumor necrosis factor (TNF)-α, transforming growth factor β, prostaglandin E2, and hormones act together to control osteoclasts. Osteoblasts arise from pluripotent mesenchymal stem cells that can also differentiate into chondrocytes, myotubes, and adipocytes.[2]

During the remodeling process a previously quiescent bone surface is activated by unknown signals that attract osteoclast precursors from the circulation to the skeleton, where they join together and form multinucleated cells. Osteocytes are believed to play an important role in initiating bone remodeling by transmitting local signals to osteoblasts and osteoclasts on bone surfaces via a canalicular system.[3] Once formed, these multinucleated preosteoclasts attach to the bone surface, differentiate, and begin to resorb bone matrix, creating bone resorption pits. Once completed, resorption is associated with apoptosis of the osteoclasts and a reversal phase during which cells including preosteoblasts migrate to the surface of the bone. Mature osteoblasts

The author discloses that she is a consultant, is a member of the speakers' bureau, and has performed clinical trials for Amgen, the manufacturer of denosumab.
Division of Rheumatology, David Geffen School of Medicine, University of California, Los Angeles, CA, USA
* 18102 Irvine Boulevard #104, Tustin, CA 92780.
E-mail address: rkdmail@sbglobal.net

direct the formation of new bone matrix and regulate its mineralization. This phase is followed by the apoptosis of osteoblasts and the incorporation of these cells into the bone as osteocytes or their transformation into bone surface lining cells.

Postmenopausal osteoporosis is a condition of acceleration of the bone remodeling rate. After menopause each remodeling cycle leads to a net loss of bone, due to a small deficiency in the amount of new bone that is formed compared with the amount of old bone that is removed. This small deficit in bone formation can result in trabecular perforations that occur during the resorptive phase, leading to a loss of bone surface on which osteoblasts can form new bone.[4] Inhibition of bone remodeling has therefore become a major target for therapies that treat postmenopausal osteoporosis. This class of therapies includes estrogen, bisphosphonates, calcitonin, selective estrogen receptor modulators or estrogen agonist/antagonists, and denosumab.

THE ROLE OF OSTEOPROTEGERIN/RANKL/RANK IN BONE BIOLOGY

Breakthroughs in the understanding of osteoclast differentiation and activation came from the analysis of a family of biologically related TNF/TNF-like proteins: osteoprotegerin (OPG), receptor activator of nuclear factor (NF) κB (RANK), and RANK ligand (RANKL), all of which regulate osteoclast function. RANKL is expressed on the surface of marrow stromal cells, activated T cells, and precursors of bone-forming osteoblasts.[5] RANKL accelerates osteoclastogenesis when it binds to its receptor RANK on osteoclast precursor cells to enhance NF-κB and other signaling pathways. This binding of RANKL to RANK promotes osteoclast formation, activation, and survival. OPG is a soluble cytokine receptor that competes with RANK to bind RANKL, thus sequestering RANKL and neutralizing its effects. Thus OPG, which is produced by osteoblasts, is a natural decoy receptor for RANKL.

The OPG/RANKL/RANK system plays a significant role in postmenopausal osteoporosis. Postmenopausal women express higher levels of RANKL on marrow stromal cells or lymphocytes than premenopausal women or postmenopausal women taking estrogen.[6] RANKL expression is inversely correlated with serum levels of 17β-estradiol and positively correlated with levels of bone resorption markers.[6] The activity of c-jun N-terminal kinase, an intracellular signal following RANK activation, can be suppressed by 17β-estradiol.[7]

Glucocorticoid-induced osteoporosis is also characterized by increased bone resorption initially followed by decreased bone formation. Glucocorticoid exposure increases RANKL expression, inhibits OPG production by osteoblasts, and suppresses OPG levels.[8,9] The OPG/RANKL/RANK system also plays an active role in posttransplant osteoporosis through the use of immunosuppressive drugs.[10] Although levels of soluble RANKL and OPG can be measured in the serum, these values can be influenced by age, renal function, and vascular disease[11]; thus measurement of soluble RANKL and OPG for diagnosis, risk stratification, or therapeutic monitoring of bone-related diseases is not recommended for routine clinical practice.

TREATMENT IMPLICATIONS

Restoring a balanced RANKL/OPG ratio or blocking RANK binding should prevent osteoclast activation and bone resorption. In a study by Bekker and colleagues,[12] a single subcutaneous dose of OPG caused rapid and sustained inhibition of bone resorption as indicated by bone resorption markers. The injection was well tolerated. It is evident from this study that OPG could potentially have clinical applications as a new antiresorptive therapy to treat osteoporosis. OPG, however, is a fairly large protein, which can be difficult to administer in ways other than by injection, and its short half-life would require monthly dosing to maintain consistent suppression of bone resorption. Another potential risk with OPG is the formation of anti-OPG antibodies, which could cross-react with endogenous OPG, neutralizing its activity. Anti-OPG antibodies were seen in one patient in this study. No negative effects were seen clinically, but safety concerns could arise with chronic dosing. Given these limitations, a RANKL inhibitor with a longer half-life and less immunogenicity would be preferable. Monoclonal antibodies have significantly longer half-lives than Fc fusion proteins (such as the OPG injection), so a fully human monoclonal antibody directed against human RANKL was developed.[13] This monoclonal antibody, denosumab, inhibits RANKL with a high specificity, mimicking the effects of OPG on RANKL (**Fig. 1**). Denosumab is classified as a highly specific molecule because it does not bind to other members of the TNF family, including TNF-α, TNF-β, TNF-related apoptosis-inducing ligand (TRAIL), or CD40 ligand.[14] Denosumab has been investigated as a therapy to treat women with postmenopausal osteoporosis and to treat men and women undergoing sex hormone ablation therapy for cancer, to prevent loss of bone mass related to these therapies.

DENOSUMAB (PROLIA)
Phase 1 Single-Dose, Dose-Escalation Study

A single-dose, placebo-controlled, dose-escalation study with denosumab in postmenopausal women was performed to determine its safety and antiresorptive effect in bone.[15] The mean age ranged from 54 to 63 years and subjects were 7 to 15 years postmenopausal. Bone density was not measured during the study.

After a single subcutaneous dose of denosumab, there was a dose-dependent decrease in bone turnover as reflected by changes in urinary N-terminal telopeptide (NTX)/creatinine and serum NTX. At the higher doses of denosumab, decreases in urine NTX/creatinine were observed as early as 12 hours after the dose: −46% in the placebo group and −77% in the denosumab group. This result suggested that

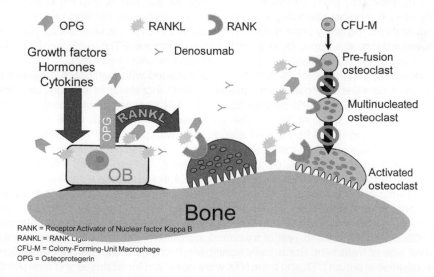

Fig. 1. RANKL Antibody/RANKL: activation of osteoclasts. (*Adapted from* Boyle WJ, Simonet WS, Lacey DL. Osteoclast differentiation and activation. Nature 2003;423:337; with permission.)

mature and active osteoclastic activity was inhibited almost immediately. The maximum urinary NTX/creatinine reduction was observed at 2 weeks in the 0.01, 0.03, 0.3, and 1.0 mg/kg groups, at 1 month in the 0.1 mg/kg group, and at 3 months in the 3.0 mg/kg group. Therefore, little if any osteoclastic activity remained while denosumab was in the circulation, but this treatment effect was reversible, as indicated by a return toward baseline levels of urinary NTX/creatinine at 2 months in the 0.01 and 0.03 mg/kg groups, at 4 months in the 0.1 mg/kg group, at 6 months in the 0.3 mg/kg group, and at 9 months in the 1.0 and 3.0 mg/kg groups. The serum NTX data confirmed the findings seen with urinary NTX/creatinine. The bone alkaline phosphatase levels remained close to baseline levels in all groups until about 2 weeks post dose, then demonstrated a dose-dependent decrease; this was expected, as denosumab does not primarily interfere with osteoblastic activity. The reduction in levels of markers of bone resorption and formation suggests that denosumab reduced the activation frequency (or birth rate) of BMUs, the cellular units responsible for bone turnover.

None of the subjects discontinued the study because of an adverse event. The incidence of reported infectious events was similar across groups (33% in the placebo group and 38% in the denosumab group overall, with no apparent dose-dependent increase). Partial inhibition of early T-lymphocyte and B-lymphocyte development has been seen in RANKL-deficient mice.[16] There was no clinically significant effect on lymphocyte counts overall (CD3), T cells (CD4, CD8, CD56), or B cells (CD20) in this study. No antidenosumab antibodies were seen in this study.

Phase 2 Study of Postmenopausal Women with Low Bone Mineral Density

This study was performed to assess the efficacy and safety of denosumab through 24 months in postmenopausal women with low bone mineral density (BMD) including those with both osteopenia and osteoporosis.[17] It was a randomized, dose-ranging, placebo-controlled, and active-controlled study involving 8 double-blind treatment groups and one open-label treatment group (alendronate). Participants received one of the following: placebo subcutaneously every 3 months, denosumab 6, 14, or 30 mg subcutaneously every 3 months, denosumab 14, 60, 100, or 210 mg subcutaneously every 6 months alternating with placebo to maintain the blinding or open-label alendronate 70 mg orally once weekly. BMD, bone turnover markers, serum chemistries, hematology assessments, intact parathyroid hormone (PTH) levels, serum denosumab levels, and denosumab-neutralizing antibodies were measured.

Denosumab treatment for 24 months was associated with significant increases in BMD from baseline compared with placebo. BMD increases in the lumbar spine ranged from 4.13% to 8.89% compared with a −1.18% change from baseline in the placebo group ($P<.001$). At 24 months, all doses of denosumab were associated with significant increases from baseline compared with placebo ($P<.001$) for BMD of the total hip, distal one-third radius and total body. When the active treatment groups were compared at 24 months, denosumab treatment was associated with similar or greater increases in BMD than alendronate at all 4 skeletal sites with the exception of the 14-mg 6-month dose. Denosumab treatment maintained reductions in serum C-terminal telopeptide (CTX) and urine NTX compared with placebo ($P<.001$) and reductions in bone-specific alkaline phosphatase (BSAP) compared with placebo ($P<.002$) during the second year of treatment, consistent with reductions seen during the first year of treatment. Statistically significant ($P<.001$) median percent reductions from baseline in serum CTX and urine NTX were observed for all doses and time points except the 14-mg 6-month dose group, for which values approached baseline levels at the time points just before the next denosumab dose (**Fig. 2**).

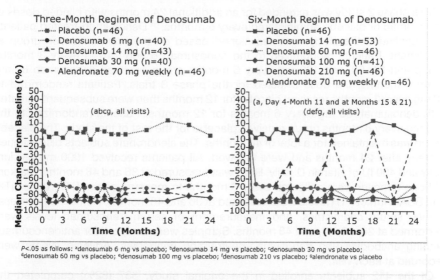

Fig. 2. Denosumab lowered serum C-telopeptide. (*From* Lewiecki EM, Miller PD, McClung MR, et al. Two-year treatment with denosumab (AMG 162) in a randomized phase 2 study of postmenopausal women with low bone mineral density. J Bone Miner Res 2007;22: 1832–41; with permission.)

The percentage of subjects who experienced adverse events during the 2-year study period was generally similar among the placebo, denosumab, and alendronate groups. Upper respiratory tract infection was the most common adverse event in the denosumab group (17.4% placebo, 24.2% denosumab, 23.9% alendronate). The incidences of hypertension and urinary tract infection were greater in the denosumab group than in the placebo group. Serious adverse events were reported in 4 (8.7%), 42 (13.4%), and 6 (13.0%) of subjects in the placebo, denosumab, and alendronate groups, respectively. Six cases of serious adverse events of infections associated with hospitalization were observed in the denosumab group (2 cases each of diverticulitis and pneumonia and 1 case each of atypical pneumonia and labyrinthitis). These events were common community-acquired infections that were successfully treated with standard antibiotics during uncomplicated hospital courses. The small study size and the disproportionately greater number of subjects assigned to denosumab treatment make it difficult to determine the clinical relevance of these small differences observed among treatment groups for some of the adverse events. Analysis by exposure-adjusted rates revealed that rates of occurrence of adverse events among all treatment groups did not increase with extended time of exposure to the study drug. Two subjects had transient, nonneutralizing antibodies to denosumab in the first 12 months. No neutralizing antibodies to denosumab were observed during the first or second year of treatment.

These changes in BMD and bone resorption markers with denosumab use over a 2-year period were consistent with a reduction in osteoclast-mediated bone resorption through inhibition of RANKL. Reversal in the suppression of bone turnover markers at the end of each dosing interval with the lower dose of denosumab suggested a reversible effect of denosumab on osteoclasts and their precursors. These results suggested that further study of denosumab to treat postmenopausal osteoporosis was warranted.

This phase 2 study was extended for an additional 24 months with blinded doses of denosumab or placebo administered every 6 months.[18] Denosumab-treated patients who continued the study were reassigned based on their randomization group at enrollment. Patients randomized to the denosumab 6 and 14 mg every 3 months group and 14, 60, and 100 mg every 6 months group received denosumab 60 mg every 6 months, the dose selected for the phase 3 trials. Patients randomized to 30 mg every 3 months received placebo for 12 months then were subsequently treated with denosumab 60 mg every 6 months for 12 months. Patients randomized to the 210 mg every 6 months group received placebo for the rest of the study. The placebo group was maintained for a total of 48 months. The alendronate subjects discontinued therapy after 24 months and were followed. All patients received 1000 mg calcium daily and 400 IU of vitamin D daily. BMD was measured at 36 and 48 months. Markers of bone turnover were collected every 6 months to measure serum CTX, urine NTX, and BSAP. Intact PTH levels were assessed at 36 and 48 months. Hematology assessments, serum chemistries, and measurement of serum denosumab levels were performed at 30, 36, 42, and 48 months. Samples were analyzed for antidenosumab-binding antibodies and denosumab-neutralizing antibodies. Adverse events were recorded at each visit.

Of the 412 subjects enrolled in the original study, 337 (82%) completed the 24-month study, 307 (75%) of these subjects entered the extension, and 262 (64%) of the original cohort completed the 48 months of treatment. Discontinuation was balanced among groups, with the most common reason for discontinuation being withdrawal of consent (94/412 = 23%). Increases in BMD reached similar levels for all groups that switched to 60 mg every 6 months. Almost all of the subjects who received denosumab treatment for 48 months had increases in BMD (greater than 0%) at the lumbar spine (97.4%) and total hip (95.5%) whereas most subjects in the placebo group lost BMD at these sites (72.4% and 82.8%, respectively).

As mentioned previously, markers of bone turnover (serum CTX, urine NTX, and BSAP) were rapidly reduced by denosumab treatment and remained substantially decreased over the entire 48 months of the study. During the last 24 months of the study, markers of bone turnover were measured at 6-month intervals just before the next dose, which corresponded to the nadir of the serum denosumab levels. Only a small percentage of denosumab-treated patients ($\leq$6.8%) had serum CTX levels below the quantifiable limit of the assay (0.049 ng/mL) at 30, 36, 42, and 48 months. In the denosumab 210 mg every 6 months treatment group that discontinued therapy at 24 months, the levels of serum CTX and urine NTX returned to values near baseline and were not significantly different from placebo.

For the 30 mg every 3 months group that was assigned to placebo at 24 months for 12 months and then retreated with denosumab 60 mg every 6 months for 12 months, BMD increased to a similar degree to that observed after initial denosumab treatment. By month 48, the lumbar spine BMD had increased 9% and the total hip BMD had increased 3.9% from baseline. Markers of bone turnover rapidly decreased to values below baseline after retreatment with denosumab. At 42 and 48 months, values of markers of bone turnover were similar to those of the continuous treatment groups.

To further evaluate the effect of discontinuing denosumab therapy on bone remodeling, data for the 210 mg and 30 mg every 3 months treatment group were combined because both of these groups stopped denosumab at the end of the 24 months. Despite the increase in serum CTX levels after discontinuation of denosumab, most patients (42/62 = 68%) had serum CTX levels within the range for postmenopausal women as defined by the assay manufacturer (mean = 0.439 ng/mL). At month 48, all except one subject had serum CTX levels below the upper range limit (1.351 ng/mL) for this assay. The clinical consequences of the increase in levels of markers of bone turnover and the decrease in BMD after discontinuing denosumab therapy are unknown.

Most patients experienced an adverse event over the 48 months of the study. The most common adverse events reported were upper respiratory tract infections, arthralgia, and back pain. Serious adverse events were reported by 10.9% (5/46) subjects in the placebo group, 17.8% (56/314) subjects in the denosumab group, and 17.4% (8/46) subjects in the alendronate group. Overall, the incidence of malignancy was balanced among the treatment groups: 4.3% (2/46) in the placebo group, 4.8% (15/314) in the denosumab group, and 4.3% (2/46) in the alendronate group. The overall incidence of infections was similar for all treatment groups: 67.4% (31/46) for placebo, 66.2% (208/314) for denosumab, and 69.6% (32/46) for alendronate. None of the placebo or alendronate-treated patients developed infections requiring hospitalization; however, 3.2% (10/314) of the denosumab-treated patients did. All of the infections were common community-acquired infections, and no opportunistic infections were reported. Infections were treated with standard antibiotics and hospitalizations were uncomplicated. Four deaths (gastric cancer, adenocarcinoma, brain cancer, and cerebral vascular accident) occurred in the 314 denosumab-treated patients. No deaths occurred in the smaller placebo or alendronate groups. No patients experienced clinically relevant changes in chemistry or hematology values. No patient experienced symptomatic hypocalcemia, and no patients developed neutralizing antibodies to denosumab.

This study was not powered to assess reduction in fracture risk with denosumab compared with placebo or alendronate. Clinical fractures were reported as adverse events. Clinical fractures occurred in 10.9% (5/46) of the placebo subjects, 10.5% (33/314) of the denosumab subjects, and 6.5% (3/46) of the alendronate subjects. There was no increase in fracture incidence in the groups that discontinued denosumab treatment, but the size of these groups was small and the follow-up period was short. Further studies need to be performed to determine if a limited period of increased bone remodeling after discontinuing denosumab therapy increases the risk of fracture.

This study[17] was extended for an additional 4 years to permit continued evaluation of efficacy and safety of continuous denosumab exposure for up to 8 years. An interim analysis from that extension has been published, representing up to 6 years of exposure to denosumab.[19] BMD was measured at the lumbar spine, total hip, femoral neck, and one-third radius at study entry and years 5 and 6. Bone turnover markers (serum CTX, urine NTX, and serum BSAP) were measured after an overnight fast and before the next denosumab dose, and an additional draw for CTX was performed at 1 month after the dose in year 1 and year 5 of the extension study. All patients in the extension study received denosumab 60 mg every 6 months (including the placebo and off-alendronate groups) but were grouped for analysis purposes according to the treatment regimens received during the 48-month study. Because this extension study did not have a control group, the data from the original 48-month study served as the comparator for both efficacy and safety measures.

Two hundred subjects entered the extension study and 178 completed the 6-year assessment. Six years of continuous treatment was associated with mean BMD increases of 13.3%, 6.1%, and 5.6% at the lumbar spine, total hip, and femoral neck. Even the subjects who had not received continuous denosumab treatment showed similar increases in BMD at the lumbar spine, total hip, and femoral neck. All subjects demonstrated continued increases in BMD over a 6-year period, without evidence of a plateau, which is not seen with other antiresorptive therapies. The mechanism to explain this finding is not known, but at least 3 hypotheses have been discussed. One hypothesis is that denosumab closes the remodeling space and prolongs remodeling with subsequent increases in mineralization over time. Another is that denosumab causes greater reductions in bone resorption and longer remodeling time compared with alendronate, independent of bone surface available for remodeling, resulting in fewer new bone remodeling units and simultaneous filling-in of preexisting resorption cavities. The third hypothesis suggests that the increase in CTX seen at the end of the dosing interval allows for some degree of remodeling, which mineralizes after the next denosumab dose.

At year 6, serum CTX remained below the 48-month study baseline with a median reduction of 54.8% compared with baseline. To determine the differential effects of short-term and long-term denosumab therapy on the magnitude of reduction in CTX, the CTX values at 1 month after dose in years 1 and 5 were compared with those at baseline in the 48-month study, which showed median reductions of 89.3% and 91.2%, respectively. Median reductions in CTX just before the next dose for these intervals were 72.1% in year 1 and 47.5% in year 5. All subjects demonstrated reductions in CTX and BSAP, independent of prior treatment assignment. Both markers of bone turnover remained within the premenopausal reference range when measured in the study extension. The gradual increase in CTX over time with continuous denosumab exposure may reflect discrete changes in the degree of RANKL expression. Further investigation is needed to test this hypothesis.

One hundred and sixty-six subjects (83%) reported at least one adverse event. The 3 most common adverse events of upper respiratory infection (13.5%), arthralgia (11.5%), and back pain (9%) were similar to those seen in the 48 month study. Twenty-six subjects (13%) experienced a serious adverse event. Malignancy was reported in 3.5% of subjects: 1 metastatic cancer of unknown origin, 1 breast carcinoma in situ, 1 breast cancer, 2 lung cancers, and 1 colon cancer. Three infections were associated with hospitalization: pneumonia, endocarditis with staphylococcal septicemia, and diverticulitis. Three deaths occurred during the extension study: one due to unknown causes, one due to liver cancer, and one due to chronic obstructive pulmonary disease. Nine subjects suffered at least one fracture during the extension study. Sites of the fractures included fibula, foot, rib, humerus, hand, radius, thoracic spine, and tibia. There were no reports of delayed fracture healing or nonunion of fractures. No clinically relevant changes in blood chemistries were observed. No subjects developed antibodies to denosumab during the extension study. Thus, the overall safety profile in this ongoing study extension did not change over time. Denosumab was well tolerated and effective through 6 years of continuous treatment.

Phase 3 Study of Postmenopausal Women with Low Bone Mass (DEFEND)

The Denosumab Fortifies Bone Density (DEFEND) trial evaluated the efficacy and safety of denosumab over a 2-year period compared with a placebo control in a population of postmenopausal women with low bone density but not osteoporosis.[20] This trial was a 2-year randomized, double-blind, placebo-controlled study performed in North America. An extension phase is ongoing. The primary end point was percent change in lumbar spine BMD at 24 months. Additional end points were percent change in volumetric BMD of the distal radius by quantitative computed tomography (QCT); percent change in BMD for the total hip, one-third radius, and total body; hip structural analysis; percent change in markers of bone turnover; and safety. Subjects were randomly assigned to receive denosumab subcutaneously at a dose of 60 mg every 6 months or placebo. Randomization was stratified by time since onset of menopause, that is, less than or equal to 5 years or more than 5 years.

A total of 332 subjects were enrolled in the study. Time since onset of menopause was 5 years or less in 162 subjects and more than 5 years in 170 subjects. Completion rate was 86%, with withdrawal of consent as the most common reason for study discontinuation. The lumbar spine BMD increase for the denosumab group overall was 6.5% at month 24 compared with −0.6% for placebo. BMD increased rapidly with significant increases seen as early as 1 month compared with placebo. The BMD increases at 24 months for the denosumab group overall were 3.4% at the total hip, 1.4% at the one-third radius, and 2.4% for the total body compared with changes of −1.1%, −2.1%, and −1.4%, respectively, in the placebo group overall. QCT analysis of the distal forearm showed that denosumab significantly ($P<.01$) increased total volumetric BMD at the distal forearm for both strata and the strata combined compared with placebo at 24 months. Denosumab treatment significantly increased BMD, cross-sectional area, cross-sectional moment of inertia, section modulus, and average cortical thickness relative to placebo at all 3 cross sections but had no significant effect on the outer diameter. These results suggest that the modulation of bone remodeling by denosumab may result in a pattern of effects on cortical bone that may be beneficial.[21] Whether this observation will result in greater fracture reduction in cortical bone compared with other antiresorptive therapy is unknown.

Markers of bone resorption were rapidly reduced by denosumab treatment. Levels of C-terminal telopeptide of collagen type I (CTX-I) reached a nadir at 1 month with a median reduction of 89% from baseline in the denosumab treatment group overall, compared with a 3% decrease in the placebo group overall ($P<.0001$). Continued suppression of CTX-I was maintained on denosumab treatment, with reductions from baseline of 63% to 88% observed at the remaining study visits. Denosumab treatment also reduced levels of the bone formation marker, procollagen type 1 amino-terminal propeptide (P1NP), which declined more gradually than CTX-I.

The overall incidence of adverse events during the 24 months was similar between the placebo and denosumab groups. The most common adverse events in both treatment groups were arthralgia, nasopharyngitis, and back pain, with more subjects on denosumab reporting sore throat and rashes. Serious adverse events were reported in 9 subjects in the placebo group (5.5%) and 18 subjects in the denosumab group (11%) ($P = .074$). The higher incidence of serious adverse events in the denosumab group was primarily due to a larger number of subjects who had infections treated as hospital inpatients (8 denosumab subjects, 1 placebo subject). The overall incidence of infections reported as adverse events was balanced between the two groups (61% placebo subjects, 60% denosumab subjects). The types of infections reported in the hospitalized subjects were common infections such as pneumonia, diverticulitis, sepsis, pyelonephritis, cellulitis, appendicitis, urinary tract infections in the denosumab subjects, and lobar pneumonia in the placebo subject. No opportunistic infections were seen. Hospitalizations were characterized by uncomplicated courses and successful treatment with standard antibiotics. Malignancies were reported in 1 subject in the placebo group (B-cell lymphoma) and in 4 subjects in the denosumab group (breast carcinoma in situ, mycosis fungoides, uterine cancer, and ovarian cancer) ($P = .215$). No deaths occurred during the study. Three subjects (2%) in the placebo group and 2 subjects (1%) in the denosumab group developed nonneutralizing antidenosumab antibodies. Data from this study suggested that denosumab administered subcutaneously at a dose of 60 mg every 6 months was suitable for further evaluation of its ability to reduce osteoporotic-related fractures.

The purpose of the 2-year extension study of this phase 3 trial was to determine the effects of denosumab discontinuation on bone density and bone turnover markers.[22] One hundred and twenty-eight subjects discontinued denosumab and 128 continued on placebo. After discontinuation of denosumab, levels of CTX increased to levels 40% to 60% above pretreatment values for the first 6 months of the extension study, then gradually returned to baseline by month 48 (month 24 of the extension study). Bone density also decreased in the off-treatment group, reaching baseline BMD after 12 months off-denosumab and remaining stable over the next 12 months. Thus, this study demonstrated reversibility of bone turnover markers and BMD on discontinuation of denosumab after 24 months.

Fractures in this study were captured as adverse events, as the extension study was not powered to evaluate fracture risk reduction. The incidence of nonvertebral fractures during the off-treatment study period was placebo 4 (3.1%) and off-treatment denosumab 4 (3.1%). One vertebral fracture occurred in the denosumab off-treatment group. It can be postulated that even though BMD decreased and CTX levels increased off-treatment, the fact that there was not an increase in fractures during this period of time and that the BMD and CTX values returned to baseline suggests that this 2-year off-treatment period has no long-term consequences.

Phase 3 Study of Denosumab for Prevention of Fractures in Postmenopausal Women with Osteoporosis

The Fracture Reduction Evaluation of Denosumab in Osteoporosis Every 6 Months (FREEDOM) trial was an international, randomized, placebo-controlled trial comparing subcutaneous injections of either 60 mg of denosumab or placebo every 6 months for 36 months.[23] The primary end point was new vertebral fracture. Secondary end points were time to the first nonvertebral fracture and time to the first hip fracture. Randomization was stratified according to 5-year age groups. Women were eligible for inclusion if they were between the age of 60 and 90 years with a BMD T-score of less than −2.5 but greater than −4 at the lumbar spine or total hip, and did not have any severe or no more than 2 moderate vertebral fractures.

A total of 7876 women were enrolled in the study, 3935 in the placebo group and 3933 in the denosumab group. Baseline characteristics were similar between the two study groups. The mean BMD T-scores were −2.8 at the lumbar spine, −2.2 at the femoral neck, and −1.9 at the total hip. Approximately 24% of women had a prevalent vertebral fracture. Eighty-two percent (6478/7868) of subjects completed all 36 months of the study and 76% (5979/7868) received all of the injections.

The 36-month incidence of new radiographic vertebral fractures was 7.2% (264/3691) in the placebo group and 2.3% (86/3702) in the denosumab group, representing a 68% relative risk reduction (P<.001). The reduction in risk was similar during each year of the trial (**Fig. 3**). The reduction in clinical vertebral fractures (69%) and multiple new vertebral fractures (61%) was similar (P<.001 for both comparisons). Denosumab reduced the risk of nonvertebral fracture, with a cumulative incidence of 8% in the placebo group compared with 6.5% in the denosumab group for a relative risk reduction of 20% (hazard ratio 0.80; 95% confidence interval [CI] 0.67–0.95; P = .01). Denosumab also decreased the risk of hip fracture, with a cumulative incidence of 1.2% in the placebo group compared with 0.7% in the denosumab group for a relative risk reduction of 40% (hazard ratio 0.60; 95% CI 0.37–0.97; P = .04). After 36 months compared with placebo, denosumab was associated with a relative increase in BMD of 9.2% (95% CI 8.2–10.1) at the lumbar spine and 6% (95% CI 5.2–6.7) at the total hip. Denosumab decreased serum CTX levels by 86% at 1 month, by 72% at 6 months before treatment was readministered, and by 72% at 36 months compared with placebo. Levels of P1NP were 18%, 50%, and 76% compared with placebo at the same time points.

There were no significant differences in the total incidence of adverse events, serious adverse events, or discontinuation of study treatment due to adverse events between subjects who received denosumab or received placebo. There were no significant differences in the overall incidence of cardiovascular events, cancer, or

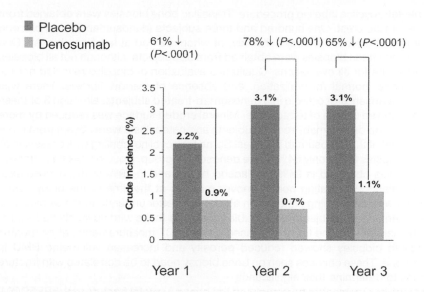

Fig. 3. FREEDOM: vertebral fracture risk reduction. (*Data from* Cummings SR, Martin JS, McClung MR, et al. Denosumab for prevention of fractures in postmenopausal women with osteoporosis. N Engl J Med 2009;368:756–65.)

infection, either adverse or serious adverse. Seventy subjects (1.8%) died in the denosumab group and 90 (2.3%) in the placebo group (*P* = .08). Four opportunistic infections were seen in the denosumab group and 3 in the placebo group. Twelve subjects (0.3%) in the denosumab group reported serious adverse events of cellulitis compared with 1 subject (*P* = .002) in the placebo group, although there were no differences in the overall incidence of cellulitis with 36 (0.9%) in the placebo group and 47 (1.2%) in the denosumab group. There was no difference in the number of subjects who experienced injection site reactions between the denosumab and placebo groups. No cases of osteonecrosis of the jaw occurred in either group. Delayed fracture healing was reported in 4 subjects in the placebo group and in 2 subjects in the denosumab group. One case of nonunion of a humerus fracture was reported in the placebo group. There were 3 fractures of the femoral shaft in the placebo group (0.1%) and none in the denosumab group. Three events of hypocalcemia (0.1%) occurred in the placebo group and none were reported in the denosumab group. Neutralizing antibodies to denosumab did not develop in any subject. Adverse events occurring in at least 2% of subjects and with a significant difference between groups included eczema (3% of subjects in the denosumab group and 1.7% in the placebo group [*P*<.001]), falls not associated with a fracture (4.5% of subjects in the denosumab group and 5.7% in the placebo group [*P* = .02]), and flatulence (2.2% of subjects in the denosumab group and 1.4% in the placebo group [*P* = .008]).

A subset of patients in the FREEDOM trial underwent bone biopsies.[24] Bone biopsies provide an assessment of the quality of bone tissue, including mineralization and microstructure, an essential safety parameter. In addition, histomorphometry provides a direct assessment of bone remodeling. Micro computed tomography (microCT) was performed on some of the biopsies, allowing assessment of bone microarchitecture and density in 3 dimensions. Subjects underwent bone biopsies in the 56 days before the month-24 and/or month-36 visits. All subjects scheduled for biopsy followed a double-tetracycline labeling procedure. Transiliac bone biopsies were obtained from the anterior iliac crest. One hundred and three subjects (denosumab 52 and placebo 51) enrolled in the bone biopsy substudy, of whom 92 had at least one biopsy. One hundred and fifteen biopsies were obtained from 92 subjects, although not all biopsies were adequate for all evaluations. Qualitative evaluation of biopsies revealed normal lamellar bone, normal mineralization, and absence of marrow fibrosis. There was a qualitative absence of osteoid in 5 denosumab-treated subjects, although 3 of these biopsies showed uptake of tetracycline. Mineral eroded surface was reduced by more than 80% in the denosumab-treated subjects and osteoclasts were absent from more than one-half of the denosumab biopsies. Some tetracycline labeling was present in all placebo biopsies but in only 64% of the denosumab group. Double labeling in trabecular bone was observed in 94% of placebo bones and in 19% of the denosumab-treated patients. Circulating bone turnover markers at the time of the biopsy were compared with the labeling status in an attempt to better understand the significance of the absent labels. Subjects with double labels and those with no labels had similar levels of markers of bone turnover. Based on microCT measurements, at 24 months denosumab biopsies showed reduced porosity and increased volumetric BMD in cortical bone. These changes seen on bone biopsy need to be correlated with fracture reduction to determine their significance.

A total of 4550 subjects who completed the phase 3 pivotal fracture trial (FREEDOM) enrolled into a 7-year open-label, single-arm extension study to evaluate the long-term efficacy and safety of denosumab.[25] All subjects in the extension study receive denosumab 60 mg every 6 months regardless of treatment assignment in the pivotal fracture trial. The primary end point of the extension study is to assess the safety and tolerability of up to 10 years of denosumab administration. Secondary end points of the extension study include changes in bone turnover, changes in bone density, and incidence of new vertebral and new nonvertebral fractures. During the extension study, denosumab treatment continued to significantly increase BMD in the lumbar spine and total hip in years 4 and 5. Adverse events reported in the denosumab-treated subjects in years 4 and 5 were similar to those observed in the initial 3 years of the pivotal fracture trial. No significant increase in malignancies was observed in the extension study. The rate of overall infection and serious infection in the extension study was similar to that observed in the 3-year pivotal fracture study (**Table 1**).

Table 1
Summary of adverse events through 5 years: rate per 100 patient-years

	Pivotal Phase 3 Fracture Trial		Extension Study
	Placebo n = 3883 Rate (Event)	Denosumab n = 3879 Rate (Event)	Denosumab-Treated Subjects During Years 4 and 5 n = 2343 Rate (Event)
All adverse events	237	235	180
Infectious	40.2	39.8	33.3
Eczema	0.7	1.3	1.1
Hypocalcemia	<0.1 (3)	0	<0.1 (1)
Serious adverse events	16.4	17.3	15.3
Infectious	1.4	1.8	1.4
Cellulitis or erysipelas	<0.1 (1)	0.1 (13)	<0.1 (3)
Malignancies	1.8	2.0	2.1

Phase 3 Study of Transitioning from Alendronate to Denosumab (STAND)

This study was conducted in postmenopausal women previously treated with alendronate to determine the effects of transitioning directly to denosumab on BMD, markers of bone turnover, and safety compared with continuing branded alendronate therapy. It was a 12-month randomized, double-blind, double-dummy, active comparator trial[26] with the primary end point of percent change in total hip BMD from baseline to month 12. Subjects received either denosumab 60 mg subcutaneously every 6 months plus an oral placebo tablet once weekly, or a placebo injection every 6 months plus a weekly oral alendronate tablet. Subjects were postmenopausal women 55 years or older with BMD T-scores between −2.0 and −4.0 at the lumbar spine or total hip who had taken at least 6 months of alendronate therapy. BMD at the total hip increased by 1.9% (95% CI 1.61%–2.18%) at month 12 in subjects transitioned from alendronate compared with 1.05% (95% CI 0.76%–1.34%) in those subjects continuing alendronate. Superiority testing demonstrated that the BMD increase seen with denosumab at the total hip was statistically superior to the change seen with alendronate ($P<.0001$). Significantly greater increases in BMD with denosumab compared with alendronate were also observed at month 12 at the lumbar spine, femoral neck, and one-third radius. CTX-I levels decreased significantly by day 5 to 0.05 ng/mL in response to transitioning to denosumab. This reduction remained stable at months 1 and 3, followed by an attenuation of the reduction before the next dose at month 6. The incidence of serious adverse events of infections and malignancies was similar between groups. No subjects were positive for antidenosumab-binding antibodies. The study design attempted to reflect actual clinical practice when many patients are switched from one osteoporosis therapy to another. The study results demonstrated that postmenopausal women with low bone mass may be safely switched from weekly oral alendronate to every-6-month subcutaneous denosumab with incremental increases in bone density.

Phase 3 Study of Initiating Denosumab or Alendronate Therapy in Treatment-Naïve Postmenopausal Women with Low Bone Mass

The Determining Efficacy: Comparison of Initiating Denosumab vs Alendronate (DECIDE) trial was a double-blind, double-dummy, randomized trial that compared the safety and efficacy of denosumab with weekly oral branded alendronate (Fosamax) in postmenopausal women with low bone mass (T-score of −2.0 or less) with no or very limited prior bisphosphonate use.[27] The primary hypothesis was that treatment with denosumab would be noninferior to treatment with alendronate with respect to the mean percent change in the total hip BMD at 12 months. The mean percent change from baseline in BMD at the total hip was 3.5% for denosumab-treated subjects compared with 2.6% for alendronate-treated subjects ($P<.0001$). Prespecified superiority testing showed significantly greater increases in BMD in subjects treated with denosumab compared with alendronate-treated subjects at the total hip, trochanter, one-third radius, femoral neck, and lumbar spine. In denosumab-treated subjects serum CTX-I reduction was rapid, with maximal median decreases from baseline at month 1 (−89%), which was significantly greater than that observed for alendronate-treated subjects (−61%; $P<.0001$). No significant differences were observed in the overall incidence of adverse events between denosumab-treated and alendronate-treated subjects (80.9% vs 82.3%; $P = .60$). Serious adverse events were similar between denosumab-treated subjects (n = 34 [5.7%]) and alendronate-treated subjects (n = 37[6.3%]). The incidence and types of infections were similar between groups, being 221 (37.3%) in the denosumab-treated subjects and 207

(35.3%) in the alendronate-treated subjects. Serious adverse events of infection were also balanced between treatment groups, with 9 (1.5%) in the denosumab-treated subjects and 6 (1.0%) in the alendronate-treated subjects. Malignancies were reported in 6 (1.0%) denosumab and 5 (0.9%) alendronate subjects. This study demonstrated that denosumab treatment produced significantly greater increases in BMD at all measured skeletal sites compared with alendronate, and a significantly greater reduction in bone resorption. These differences, however, do not necessarily correlate with greater fracture reduction with denosumab compared with alendronate. No head-to-head fracture study comparing different osteoporosis therapies has been performed.

Study of Patient Preference and Satisfaction with Denosumab Versus Alendronate

A 34-item patient questionnaire, the Preference and Satisfaction Questionnaire (PSQ), was developed specifically to evaluate patient preference and satisfaction with two different modes and frequency of dosing for the treatment of postmenopausal bone loss: an oral tablet once weekly (alendronate) and a subcutaneous injection administered every 6 months (denosumab). Subjects enrolled in both the STAND and DECIDE studies were asked to complete the PSQ after 12 months of treatment or on study discontinuation.[28] Overall, 93% of subjects enrolled in these two trials completed at least one item of the PSQ. Demographics or baseline characteristics were very similar between subjects who took the PSQ and those who did not. Some subjects in each treatment group did not indicate a preference for either treatment (16% of denosumab-treated subjects and 17% of alendronate-treated subjects). Among subjects who reported a preference, significantly more preferred the 6-month injection (65% of the denosumab group and 63% of the alendronate) to the weekly tablet (19% for both treatment groups; $P<.0001$). Twenty percent of subjects in both treatment groups were not more satisfied with one dosing frequency over the other. Significantly more subjects in both the denosumab (64% vs 16%) and alendronate (63% vs 16%) groups were more satisfied with the dosing frequency of the 6-month injection over the weekly tablet ($P<.0001$).

An additional preference study was performed.[29] The Denosumab Adherence Preference Satisfaction Study (DAPS) compared treatment adherence, preference, and satisfaction between oral alendronate 70 mg weekly and denosumab 60 mg given subcutaneously every 6 months in postmenopausal women in a 2-year crossover design. Subjects had a BMD T-score of −2.0 to −4.0 at the lumbar spine, femoral neck, or total hip. Subjects were bisphosphonate treatment naïve and were randomized 1:1 to receive 60 mg denosumab every 6 months in year 1 followed by 70 mg alendronate weekly in year 2, or to receive treatment in the reverse order. Subjects were considered to be adherent if they received 2 denosumab injections 6 months apart or they took approximately 80% of the weekly alendronate and at least 2 alendronate tablets in the final month and returned for the final study visit. A total of 250 subjects were enrolled in the study, 126 in the denosumab/alendronate group and 124 in the alendronate/denosumab group. A total of 95 (75%) of the denosumab/alendronate and 103 (83%) of the alendronate/denosumab subjects completed the 2-year treatment period. During year 2, treatment with denosumab compared with alendronate was associated with significantly ($P<.0001$) greater adherence (92.5% vs 63.5%), compliance (93.4% vs 67.8%), and persistence (97.2% vs 71.3%) with treatment. A total of 92.4% versus 7.6% preferred denosumab injection over oral alendronate ($P<.0001$) and 91.2% versus 8.8% preferred denosumab as a long-term treatment option over oral alendronate ($P<.0001$). The study demonstrated that subjects had greater adherence, compliance, persistence, and satisfaction with denosumab treatment than with alendronate over a 2-year period. Despite the results of these two studies, to date the clinical implications of preference studies remain largely uninvestigated. It is unknown whether a preference for a semiannual injection will translate into improved long-term compliance and persistence in the community setting.

Phase 3 Study of Denosumab in Men Receiving Androgen Deprivation Therapy for Prostate Cancer

Androgen deprivation therapy (ADT) is known to increase bone resorption, decrease BMD, and increase the risk of fracture in men with prostate cancer, the risk of fracture increasing with the length of duration of ADT. The Denosumab Hormone Ablation Bone Loss Trial (HALT) was a 3-year, randomized, double-blind, multicenter center trial in which subjects were assigned to denosumab 60 mg subcutaneously every 6 months or placebo, with 734 subjects in each group.[30] The primary end point was percent change in BMD at the lumbar spine at 24 months. Key secondary end points included percent change in BMD at the femoral neck and total hip at 24 months and at all sites at 36 months, as well as the incidence of new vertebral fractures. Nine hundred and twelve patients (62.1%) completed the 36-month study. Approximately 77.9% of patients had low bone mass based on BMD T-scores with 14.7% of these having osteoporosis at baseline. At 24 months, BMD of the lumbar spine increased 5.6% in the denosumab group compared with a loss of 1% in the placebo group ($P<.001$); significant differences between the two groups were seen as early as 1 month. Denosumab therapy was also associated with significant increases in BMD at the femoral neck, total hip, and distal one-third of the radius at all time points. Subjects who received denosumab had a decreased incidence of new vertebral fractures at 12, 24, and 36 months. The cumulative incidence of new vertebral fracture was 3.9% in the placebo group and 1.5% in the denosumab group, a significant decrease of 62% (relative risk 0.38; 95% CI 0.19–0.78; $P = .006$). At 36 months, 6 months after the last dose of the study drug, levels of bone turnover markers decreased significantly in the denosumab group compared with placebo ($P<.01$). Rates of adverse events were similar between the two treatment groups. There were no cases of delayed fracture healing in either group. No cases of osteonecrosis of the jaw were reported. No neutralizing antidenosumab antibodies were detected.

A prespecified subgroup analysis was performed to evaluate the relationships between subject characteristics and the effects of denosumab on BMD at multiple skeletal sites.[31] Denosumab was found to increase BMD significantly to a similar degree, as observed in the overall study in every subgroup including older men as well as those with prevalent fractures, lower baseline BMD, and higher serum CTX and tartrate-resistant alkaline phosphatase 5b (TRAP-5b). Mean increases in BMD at each skeletal site were greatest for men with the highest levels of serum CTX and TRAP-5b at baseline.

Phase 3 Study of Denosumab in Women Receiving Adjuvant Aromatase Inhibitors for Nonmetastatic Breast Cancer

Adjuvant aromatase inhibitor (AI) therapy is known to accelerate bone loss and to increase fracture risk. In a double-blind, placebo-controlled trial women with osteopenia who were being treated with AI therapy for hormone receptor–positive breast cancer and had completed treatment (including surgery and/or radiation and chemotherapy at least 4 weeks before study entry) were randomly assigned to receive denosumab 60 mg every 6 months or placebo for a total of 4 doses.[32] A 2-year extension of this study is ongoing. Randomization was stratified by duration of prior AI therapy (≤6 months or >6 months). The primary efficacy end point was percent change from baseline in lumbar spine BMD compared with placebo at 12 months. Secondary efficacy end points included percent changes from baseline in lumbar spine BMD at 6 months, and total hip and femoral neck BMD at 6 and 12 months. A total of 252 subjects were enrolled in the study. Eighty-eight percent of patients completed 12 months of the study, with the most common reason for discontinuation being withdrawal of consent. Eighty-one percent of patients completed 24 months of the study. Baseline characteristics were generally well-balanced between treatment groups.

At 12 months, lumbar spine BMD increased by 5.5% in the denosumab group compared with the placebo group (4.8% compared with −0.7%, $P<.0001$). Increases in BMD were not influenced by duration of prior AI therapy, or whether therapy was with a nonsteroidal (anastrozole or letrozole) or steroidal (exemestane) AI therapy. Increases in lumbar spine BMD in the denosumab group were significantly different from placebo as early as 1 month ($P<.0001$). Increases in BMD were also observed at the femoral neck, total hip, one-third radius, and total body. Markers of bone turnover were rapidly reduced in the denosumab group, with serum CTX levels reaching the lowest level at 1 month, the earliest time period measured, with a median percent reduction from baseline of 91% compared with 9% in the placebo group ($P<.0001$). P1NP also decreased with denosumab therapy, with reductions of 71% to 73% between 6 and 24 months. No vertebral fractures were reported during the 24 months. The overall incidence of adverse events was similar between treatment groups, with 91% in the denosumab group and 90% in the placebo group. The most common adverse events included arthralgia, pain in the extremity, back pain, and fatigue. Rates of infections were balanced (36% for denosumab, 32% for placebo), with no apparent differences between treatment groups in types of infections. Serious adverse events involving infections treated in the hospital were reported in 3 patients (2%) in the denosumab group and in 1 patient (1%) in the placebo group. No neutralizing antidenosumab antibodies were reported.

A subgroup analysis of this study was performed to evaluate the effect of certain factors (duration and type of AI therapy, tamoxifen use, age, time since menopause, body mass index, and baseline T-score) on BMD at the lumbar spine, femoral neck, total body, and one-third radius.[33] In all subgroups, at 12 and 24 months denosumab therapy was associated with greater increases in BMD than placebo at all skeletal sites measured.

Discussion

In the studies summarized herein denosumab, a fully human monoclonal antibody, which prevents the interaction of RANKL with RANK, has been shown to increase BMD, reduce bone turnover, and reduce vertebral, nonvertebral, and hip fractures in postmenopausal women with low bone mass. Denosumab (Prolia) was recently approved by the Food and Drug Administration (FDA) for the treatment of postmenopausal women with osteoporosis at high risk for fracture, defined as a history of osteoporotic fracture, of multiple risk factors for fracture, or patients who have failed or are intolerant to other available osteoporosis therapy. The use of denosumab in patients with hypocalcemia is contraindicated. Preexisting hypocalcemia must be corrected before initiating therapy with denosumab. All patients treated with denosumab must be adequately supplemented with calcium and vitamin D. In clinical studies, patients with severe renal impairment, defined as a creatinine clearance less than 30 mL/min or receiving dialysis, were at greater risk of developing hypocalcemia.[34] In a retrospective analysis of patients from the phase 3 pivotal fracture trial (FREEDOM), similar reductions in new vertebral fractures were observed in the denosumab treatment group across different levels of renal function, although there were no subjects with a creatinine clearance of less than 15 mL/min.[35] Thus, denosumab may be considered for patients with renal insufficiency.

The studies summarized in this article also demonstrate that denosumab prevents bone loss in men with prostate cancer who are treated with ADT and in women with hormone-responsive breast cancer who are treated with AI therapy, but these are not FDA-approved indications at the present time.

In the absence of head-to-head fracture trials, it is difficult to compare the antifracture efficacy of osteoporosis therapies. Given this limitation, the antifracture efficacy of denosumab appears to be similar to that reported with teriparatide, a daily parenteral bone formation agent given for 2 years, and intravenous zoledronic acid, given yearly, with respect to vertebral, nonvertebral, and hip fractures. It is hoped that compliance and persistence will improve with less frequent dosing of therapies for postmenopausal osteoporosis, but this theory has not been proved. It is not known whether the rare adverse events seen with bisphosphonates of atypical subtrochanteric femoral fractures or osteonecrosis of the jaw will be seen with denosumab. Both classes of therapies reduce bone turnover, and treatment with denosumab has been shown to significantly suppress bone remodeling. When compared with placebo, treatment with denosumab resulted in virtually absent activation frequency and markedly reduced bone formation rates. The long-term consequences of this degree of suppression of bone remodeling are not known. The long-term consequences of suppression of bone remodeling may contribute to occurrences of osteonecrosis of the jaw (ONJ), atypical fractures, and delayed fracture healing. Although no cases of ONJ were seen in the clinical trial data that has been published in the peer-reviewed literature reviewed here, 2 adjudicated cases of ONJ occurred in subjects treated with denosumab for up to 2 years in the extension of the phase 3 pivotal fracture study. No cases of atypical fractures have been observed in the pivotal phase 3 fracture trial or in the first 2 years of the open-label extension study (up to 5 years of total treatment). Events of fracture-healing complications were reported in the phase 3 pivotal fracture study, but compared with placebo denosumab was not associated with increased occurrence of delayed fracture healing. Delayed fracture healing occurred in 6 subjects: 4 in the placebo arm (foot, clavicle, and 2 pelvic fractures) and 2 in the denosumab arm (radius/ulna and foot fracture).[25] Although it is widely believed that substantial reductions in bone remodeling over a long period of time may have adverse effects on bone strength, there are no data in human studies that document which combination of bone turnover suppression and duration of suppression is necessary to produce such adverse events. The FREEDOM trial demonstrated that substantial fracture reduction occurred in patients who had significant reductions in bone turnover for a period of 3 years. Fracture rates beyond 3 years will be monitored in the extension of the FREEDOM trial.

Another concern about long-term use of denosumab relates to its possible effects on the immune system, as RANKL is expressed on cells other than osteoclast precursors, including dendritic cells and T and B cells.[36] RANKL not only regulates osteoclastogenesis but also functions within the immune system.[37] The potential consequence of long-term RANKL inhibition on immune function was addressed in an animal model using OPG transgenic mice and rats in which RANKL is inhibited continuously throughout life. Analysis of numerous cellular, innate or adaptive, immune responses in 4- to 6-month-old transgenic mice and rats showed no differences compared with normal wild-type controls.[38,39] OPG transgenic rats in these studies had marked suppression of bone turnover and increased BMD, thus demonstrating that RANKL inhibition can cause bone turnover suppression in the absence of any measurable changes in the integrated response of the immune system. In the pivotal fracture trial, serious infections leading to hospitalization, including skin, urinary tract, abdomen, and ear infections, were reported more frequently in subjects treated with denosumab. The overall incidence of infections was similar between treatment groups, the incidence of infections resulting in death was similar in each group, and the incidence of opportunistic infections was balanced between treatment groups. Skin infections, including erysipelas and cellulitis, leading to hospitalization were reported more frequently in the denosumab-treated subjects (less than 0.1% in the placebo versus 0.4% in the denosumab-treated group). Endocarditis was reported in no placebo-treated subjects but in 3 subjects treated with denosumab. Although not statistically significant, these findings support ongoing surveillance of patients receiving denosumab, especially when the drug is used in patients on concomitant immunosuppressant medications or with impaired immune systems who are already at increased risk of infection. Patients should be advised to seek medical help if they develop signs or symptoms of serious infection after treatment with denosumab. The incidence of serious infections will continue to be monitored in the extension of the FREEDOM trial and in the denosumab (Prolia) postmarketing active safety surveillance program.

SUMMARY

Postmenopausal osteoporosis results in part from increased osteoclastic activity. The inhibition of RANKL activity by denosumab, a fully human monoclonal antibody to RANKL, increases BMD, decreases bone resorption, and reduces vertebral, nonvertebral, and hip fractures. It is hoped that use of this subcutaneous injection every 6 months will improve patient compliance and persistence compared with the weekly or monthly schedule of administration of oral, antiresorptive therapies for postmenopausal osteoporosis. Ongoing extension studies and postmarketing clinical trials will evaluate the long-term safety of this novel compound.

REFERENCES

1. Hofbauer LC, Schoppet M. Clinical implications of the osteoprotegerin RANKL/RANK system for bone and vascular diseases. JAMA 2004;292:490–5.
2. Zhao L, Huang J, Guo R, et al. Smurf 1 inhibits MSC proliferation and differentiation into osteoblasts through Jun beta degradation. J Bone Miner Res 2010; 25(6):1246–56.
3. Turner CH, Robling AG, Duncan RL, et al. Do bone cells behave like a neuronal network? Calcif Tissue Int 2002;70:435–42.
4. Compston FE, Vedi S, Kaptoge S, et al. Bone remodeling rate and remodeling balance are not co-regulated in adulthood: Implications for the use of activation frequency as an index of remodeling rate. J Bone Miner Res 2007;22:1031–6.
5. Lacey DL, Timms E, Tan HL, et al. Osteoprotegerin ligand is a cytokine that regulates osteoclast differentiation and activation. Cell 1998;93:165–76.
6. Eghbali-Fatourechi G, Khosla S, Sanyal A, et al. Role of RANK ligand in mediating increased bone resorption in early postmenopausal women. J Clin Invest 2003; 111:1221–30.
7. Shevde NK, Bendixen AC, Dienger KM. Estrogens suppress RANK ligand-induced osteoclast differentiation via a stromal cell independent mechanism involving c-Jun repression. Proc Natl Acad Sci U S A 2000;97:7829–34.
8. Hofbauer LC, Gori F, Riggs BL, et al. Stimulation of osteoprotegerin ligand and inhibition of osteoprotegerin production by glucocorticoids in human osteoblastic lineage cells. Endocrinology 1999;40:4382–9.

9. Sasaki N, Kusano E, Ando Y, et al. Glucocorticoid decreases circulating osteo-protegerin (OPG). Nephrol Dial Transplant 2001;16:479–82.
10. Fahrleitner A, Prenner G, Leb G, et al. Serum osteoprotegerin is a major determinant of bone density development and prevalent vertebral fracture status following cardiac transplantation. Bone 2003;89:180–90.
11. Browner WS, Lui LY, Cummings SR. Associations of serum osteoprotegerin levels with diabetes, stroke, bone density, fractures and mortality in elderly women. J Clin Endocrinol Metab 2001;86:631–7.
12. Bekker PJ, Holloway D, Nakanishi A, et al. The effect of a single dose of osteoprotegerin in post-menopausal women. J Bone Miner Res 2001;16:348–60.
13. Kostenuik PJ, Nguyen HQ, McCabe J, et al. Denosumab, a fully human monoclonal antibody to RANKL, inhibits bone resorption and increases BMD in knock-in mice that express chimeric (murine/human) RANKL. J Bone Miner Res 2009;24:182–95.
14. Kostenuik PJ. Osteoprotegerin and RANKL regulate bone resorption, density, geometry and strength. Curr Opin Pharmacol 2005;5:618–25.
15. Bekker PJ, Holloway DL, Rasmussen AS, et al. A single-dose placebo-controlled study of AMG-162, a fully human monoclonal antibody to RANKL, in postmenopausal women. J Bone Miner Res 2004;19(7):1059–66.
16. Kong YY, Yoshida H, Sarosi I, et al. OPGL is a key regulator of osteoclastogenesis, lymphocyte development and lymph node organogenesis. Nature 1999;397: 315–23.
17. Lewiecki EM, Miller PD, McClung MR, et al. Two-year treatment with denosumab (AMG 162) in a randomized phase 2 study of postmenopausal women with low bone mineral density. J Bone Miner Res 2007;22:1832–41.
18. Miller PD, Bolognese MA, Lewiecki EM, et al. Effect of denosumab on bone density and turnover in postmenopausal with low bone mass after long-term continued, discontinued, and restarting of therapy: a randomized blinded phase 2 clinical trial. Bone 2008;43:222–9.
19. Miller PD, Wagman RB, Peacock M, et al. Effect of denosumab on bone mineral density and biochemical markers of bone turnover: six-year results of a phase 2 clinical trial. J Clin Endocrinol Metab 2011;96(2):394–402.
20. Bone HG, Bolognese MA, Yuen CK, et al. Effects of denosumab on bone mineral density and bone turnover in postmenopausal women. J Clin Endocrinol Metab 2008;93(6):2149–57.
21. Genant HK, Engelke K, Hanley DA, et al. Denosumab improves density and strength parameters as measured by QCT of the radius in postmenopausal women with low bone mineral density. Bone 2010;47:131–9.
22. Bone HG, Bolognese MA, Yuen CK, et al. Effects of denosumab therapy and discontinuation on bone mineral density and bone turnover markers in postmenopausal women with low bone mass. J Bone Miner Res 2009;24(Suppl 1), presentation 1243.
23. Cummings SR, Martin JS, McClung MR, et al. Denosumab for prevention of fractures in postmenopausal women with osteoporosis. N Engl J Med 2009;361: 756–65.
24. Reid IR, Miller PD, Brown JP, et al. Effects of denosumab on bone histomorphometry: The FREEDOM and STAND studies. J Bone Miner Res 2010;25(10):2256–65.
25. Chupurlat R, Papapoulos S, Bone HG, et al. Long-term denosumab treatment of postmenopausal women with osteoporosis: results from the first two years of the FREEDOM extension study. American College of Rheumatology Annual Meeting. November 7–11, Atlanta, 2011. p. S903.

26. Kendler DL, Roux C, Benhamou CL, et al. Effects of denosumab on bone mineral density and bone turnover in postmenopausal women transitioning from alendronate therapy. J Bone Miner Res 2010;25:72–81.

27. Brown JP, Prince RL, Deal C, et al. Comparison of the effect of denosumab and alendronate on BMD and biochemical markers of bone turnover in postmenopausal women with low bone mass: a randomized, blinded, phase 3 trial. J Bone Miner Res 2009;24(1):153–61.

28. Kendler DL, Bessette L, Hill CD, et al. Preferences and satisfaction with a 6-month subcutaneous injection versus a weekly tablet for treatment of low bone mass. Osteoporos Int 2010;21:837–46.

29. Kendler DL, Kaur P, Siddhanti S. Open-label, crossover study evaluating the adherence, preference and satisfaction of denosumab and alendronate treatment in postmenopausal women: results of the second year of the study. J Clin Densitom 2011;14:158.

30. Smith MR, Egerdie B, Toriz NH, et al. Denosumab in men receiving androgen-deprivation therapy for prostate cancer. N Engl J Med 2009;361:745–55.

31. Smith MR, Saad F, Egerdie B, et al. Effects of denosumab on bone mineral density in men receiving androgen deprivation therapy for prostate cancer. J Urol 2009; 182:2670–2.

32. Ellis GK, Bone HG, Chlebowski R, et al. Randomized trial of denosumab in patients receiving adjuvant aromatase inhibitors for nonmetastatic breast cancer. J Clin Oncol 2008;26:4875–82.

33. Ellis KE, Bone HG, Chlebowski R. Effect of denosumab on bone mineral density in women receiving adjuvant aromatase inhibitors for non-metastatic breast cancer: subgroup analyses of a phase 3 study. Breast Cancer Res Treat 2009;118:81–7.

34. Prolia (denosumab) prescribing information. 2010.

35. Jamal SA, Ljunggren O, Stehman-Breen C, et al. The effects of denosumab on bone mineral density and vertebral fracture by level of renal function. Annual Meeting of the American Society for Bone and Mineral Research. Toronto, 2010. Presentation 1068.

36. Adami S, Gilchrist N, Lyritis G, et al. Effect of denosumab on fracture healing in postmenopausal women with osteoporosis: results from the FREEDOM trial. ECTS 2010. OP24 [online].

37. Martin TJ. Paracrine regulation of osteoclast formation and activity: milestones in discovery. J Musculoskelet Neuronal Interact 2004;4:243–53.

38. Walsh MC, Kim N, Kadono Y, et al. Osteoimmunology: interplay between the immune system and bone metabolism. Annu Rev Immunol 2006;24:33–63.

39. Stolina M, Dwyer D, Ominsky MS, et al. Rats overexpressing soluble osteoprotegerin from a prenatal stage have high bone mass but no alterations in the development of lymphoid organs or innate immune response. J Bone Miner Res 2006; 2:S153.

Assessment of Fracture Risk

Sanford Baim, MD

KEYWORDS

• Osteoporosis • Fracture • Bone density testing • FRAX

Osteoporotic fractures often result in significant disability, increased morbidity and mortality, and significant psychological and financial burden to the affected individuals, their families, and society.[1] Incident osteoporosis-related fractures in the United States are expected to increase from 2 million fractures in 2005 to a projected 3 million fractures per annum by 2025. The associated direct and indirect fracture-related costs to care for these patients are expected to increase from $17 billion to $25 billion by 2025.[2] There is a general awareness by both physicians and the lay public of the overall fracture burden of osteoporosis on society, the presence of proven therapeutic interventions approved by the US Food and Drug Administration (FDA) for the prevention and treatment of osteoporotic fractures and the necessity to effectively predict fracture events.

The diagnosis of osteoporosis is derived from the World Health Organization (WHO) central dual-energy X-ray absorptiometry (DXA) diagnostic criteria of a T-score of -2.5 or less performed at the lumbar spine, femoral neck, total hip, or one-third radius sites.[3–5] DXA bone mineral density (BMD) testing provides the clinician with an estimate of fracture risk in terms of a continuum of risk rather than a specific cut point below which most patients will fracture. It is used to calculate a patient's relative risk for any T-score or Z-score. The accuracy of BMD measurements using central DXA to predict osteoporotic fractures is comparable to the use of blood pressure measurement for prediction of stroke and is considerably superior to serum cholesterol as a predictor of myocardial infarction.[6–9] Risk stratification using BMD has been delineated by the large Marshall meta-analysis, which showed that risk of fracture increases by 1.4-fold–2.6-fold for every standard deviation (SD) decrease in BMD compared with the reference population used in the calculation (applies to T-scores or Z-scores).[7] Prediction of fracture is enhanced when using site-specific measurements such as spine BMD to predict spine fractures and femoral neck BMD to predict hip fractures.[9] Thus, for every 1 SD (equivalent to 1 T-score) decrease in spine BMD there is a 1.8-fold increased risk of spine fractures, and for every 1 SD decrease in hip BMD

The author has nothing to disclose.
Division of Endocrinology, Miller School of Medicine, University of Miami, 1400 NW 10th Avenue, Dominion Towers, Suite 809, Miami, FL 33136, USA
E-mail address: sbaim@med.miami.edu

Rheum Dis Clin N Am 37 (2011) 453–470
doi:10.1016/j.rdc.2011.07.001
0889-857X/11/$ – see front matter © 2011 Elsevier Inc. All rights reserved.

rheumatic.theclinics.com

there is a 2.6-fold increased risk of hip fractures. These measures of increased risk per SD decrease in BMD T-scores are referred to as gradients of risk. Calculation of an individual's relative risk of fracture can be performed by taking the gradient of risk at the site measured to the power of the T-score or Z-score ($GR^{T/Z}$). An individual with a T-score of -2.0 SD at the femoral neck has a relative risk of 2.6^2 or a sevenfold increased risk compared with an individual with a T-score of 0. Substitution of the Z-score for T-score provides a relative risk of an individual compared with an age, gender, and race-matched or ethnicity-matched individual with a Z-score of 0.

Large epidemiologic studies in the United States, Europe, and Australia have established that greater than 50% of osteoporosis-related fractures (low-trauma, fragility fractures) occur in patients who have a central DXA test result consistent with the WHO's criteria of osteopenia (low bone density), T-scores between -1.0 and -2.5, rather than osteoporosis, T-score less than or equal to -2.5.[10–12] The Study of Osteoporotic Fractures (SOF) found that 54% of women who sustained a hip fracture during the 5 years of the study had either osteopenia or normal bone density.[10] Together, these population-based studies indicate that incidence rates of osteoporosis-related fractures increase with increasing age and decreasing bone density, and the greatest number of low-trauma fractures occur in patients diagnosed with osteopenia.

The low sensitivity and low positive predictive values using BMD testing alone for prediction of fracture risk has led to the development of new strategies that are inclusive of risk stratification algorithms that consider independent clinical risk factors for fracture.[9] Age, personal history of fracture, prevalent fractures, parental history of osteoporosis-related fractures, glucocorticoid use, and so forth add to the gradient of risk and more accurately predict future fracture risk in the individual patient.[1,13–15] As an example, compare fracture prediction measures using BMD alone and relative risk versus calculation of absolute risk probabilities for 50-year-old and 80-year-old white women from the United States with identical T-scores of -3 but having no additional clinical risk factors for fracture other than their age disparity. Both women have the diagnosis of osteoporosis by WHO diagnostic criteria and identical 2.6^3 or an 18-fold increased relative risk of fracture compared with an individual with a T-score of 0. If both women's future fracture probability is calculated using one of the available fracture risk calculators, the risk of sustaining a fracture at the hip, spine, forearm, and humerus within the next 10 years is approximately 8% in the 50-year-old woman and 23% in the 80-year-old woman.[16] Inclusion of age as a known independent clinical risk factor results in a threefold greater risk of fracture in the older individual that is not appreciated by BMD testing alone or use of relative risk.

In absolute fracture prediction, improvement in accuracy requires an increased gradient of risk to change the performance characteristics of the test. In addition to age, gender, weight, and height (calculated body mass index [BMI]), other easily identifiable clinical risk factors (CRFs) that contribute independently to fracture risk include a personal or family history of fragility fractures, use of glucocorticoid medication, rheumatoid arthritis, cigarette smoking, excessive alcohol intake, and a variety of secondary conditions that contribute or cause fragility fractures that are inclusive of falls. The addition of non-BMD CRFs increases the performance characteristics of fracture prediction and calculation of quantitative output measures of future fracture risk. Available fracture prediction algorithms such as the WHO Fracture Risk Assessment Tool (FRAX), the Garvan Institute fracture risk calculator (Garvan), and QFractureScores (QFracture) can be seen in **Figs. 1** and **2**.[13,17–20]

The WHO Collaborating Center for Metabolic Bone Diseases developed FRAX as a robust computer-based algorithm that calculates the 10-year probability of (1) hip fractures and (2) major osteoporosis-related fractures (hip, clinical spine, humerus,

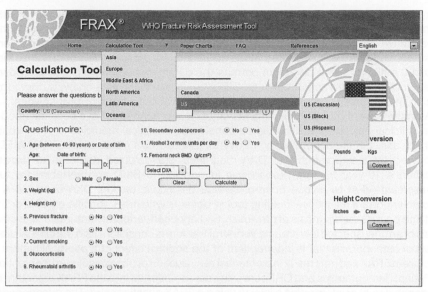

Fig. 1. FRAX with US ethnicities/races. (Available at: http://www.sheffield.ac.uk/FRAX/tool.jsp?country59.)

and forearm), with or without inclusion of femoral neck BMD.[17,20–22] FRAX calculates both fracture probabilities from easily obtained CRFs in both men and women and in the United States for Asian, black, white, and Hispanic people. Using local mortality and hip fracture rates, FRAX has been calibrated for use in more than 30 other countries.[23] FRAX calculations are based on the following variables: age, BMI, parental history of hip fracture, personal history of fragility fracture, current tobacco smoking, excessive alcohol intake, ever use of oral glucocorticoid medication, rheumatoid arthritis, and other secondary causes for osteoporosis, and takes into account the

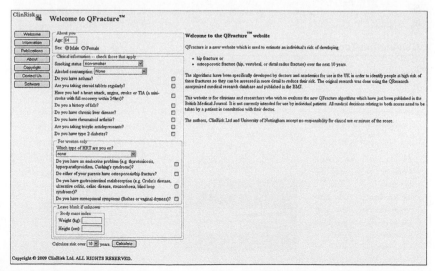

Fig. 2. *Courtesy of* ClinRisk Ltd; with permission. Available at http://www.qfracture.org/.

risk of death. The information necessary to determine the interactions between CRFs with and without BMD has been derived from a meta-analysis of 60,000 patients in 9 prospective population-based cohorts from North America, Europe, Asia, and Australia and has been validated in an additional 11 prospective cohorts involving 230,000 patients.[24] This paradigm permits the determination of the predictive power of each CRF and interaction between CRFs by using multivariate analysis, thus optimizing the accuracy of major osteoporosis-related and hip fracture probabilities.

As in the case of DXA BMD testing, FRAX 10-year probabilities have been included in many clinical guidelines and should be considered in clinical medicine as a reference point to assist in the determination of overall osteoporosis fracture risk. FRAX is FDA approved for incorporation into DXA machines' standardized printouts to provide a patient's 10-year fracture probabilities in addition to BMD and vertebral fracture assessment (VFA) as unique point-of-service diagnostic testing. DXA-based VFA is also an important adjunctive imaging tool in patients who meet specific criteria for this test and permits the diagnosis of previously undiagnosed vertebral fractures.[25] The diagnosis of an unsuspected low-trauma vertebral fracture is consistent with the clinical diagnosis of osteoporosis that is independent of the additive effect of a personal history of fracture in FRAX and may result in a potential reevaluation of pharmacologic intervention.

Patient demographics and CRF screening can be inserted into the FRAX algorithm by the technologist or interpreting clinician using a FRAX questionnaire. The questionnaire can be filled out by the patient before or at the time of bone density testing and VFA. The tool can be used online by anyone with Internet access, downloaded to an i-phone and i-pad, or used with downloaded hand-held charts.[23,26,27] Although not as accurate as FRAX with inclusion of BMD (**Fig. 3**), the algorithm is able to calculate fracture probabilities without BMD (**Fig. 4**) and is used to screen patients for further evaluation and therapeutic intervention by clinicians as part of a case-finding strategy.[1,13–15]

FRAX predicts hip-related and major osteoporosis-related fractures using BMD and 7 CRFs that contribute independently of BMD to fracture risk, and has been endorsed by the National Osteoporosis Foundation (NOF), International Society for Clinical Densitometry (ISCD), and International Osteoporosis Foundation (IOF).[1,13,28,29] FRAX

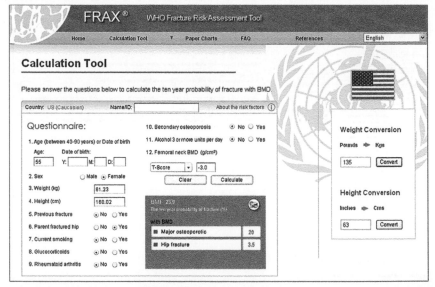

Fig. 3. FRAX with BMD. (Available at: http://www.sheffield.ac.uk/FRAX/tool.jsp?country59.)

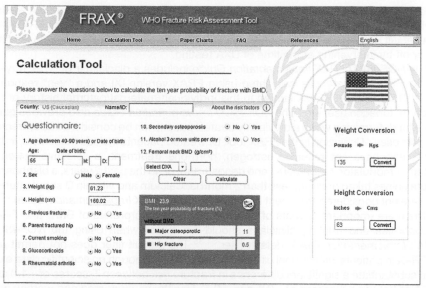

Fig. 4. FRAX without BMD. (Available at: http://www.sheffield.ac.uk/FRAX/tool.jsp?country59.)

performance characteristics have been validated in 2 long-term observational studies.[30,31] The Manitoba Bone Density Program is a long-term observational study that, independently of the FRAX cohorts, tested the performance of FRAX in 36,730 women and 2873 men using data linkage between various Canadian provincial health care databases.[30] This method permitted a direct comparison of fracture risk estimates by the Canadian FRAX tool with fractures observed during 10 years. Ten-year estimates using Kaplan-Meir curves for hip fractures in women were 2.7% (95% CI 2.1%–3.4%) compared with those predicted by the Canadian FRAX tool of 2.8%, which included BMD. In men, the observed hip fracture risk was 3.5% (95% CI 0.8%–6.2%) compared with 2.9% predicted from the Canadian FRAX tool. The observed major osteoporosis-related fractures for all women during 10 years was 12% (95% CI 10.8%–13.4%) compared with 11.1% predicted with inclusion of BMD in Canadian FRAX, whereas for all men the observed incidence of major osteoporosis-related fractures was 10.7% (95% CI 6.6%–14.9%) compared with a predicted 8.4%. Receiver operating curve analysis of the data was 0.830 (95% CI 0.815–0.846) for hip fractures and 0.694 (95% CI 0.684–0.705) for major osteoporosis-related fractures. Canadian FRAX with BMD had better performance characteristics for predicting fracture during 10 years of observation than Canadian FRAX without BMD (CRFs) or BMD alone.[30]

In 2010, the NOF and ISCD published a FRAX Implementation Guide to ensure the appropriate use of FRAX in the United States.[32,33] The *NOF-ISCD FRAX Implementation Guide* suggests that FRAX should be used in the following individuals:

a. Untreated postmenopausal women or men aged 50 years or older
b. Osteopenia or low bone mass (T-score between −1.0 and −2.5)
c. No prior hip or vertebral fracture (clinical or morphometric)
d. An evaluable hip BMD for inclusion in FRAX.

NOF-ISCD FRAX Implementation Guide software can be installed on all central DXA machines in the form of a default filter. The default filter is used to limit the use of FRAX to only individuals who meet the previously listed criteria (a–d). Central DXA testing facilities have the option to either use FRAX with the Implementation Guide FRAX filter in a default mode (filter always on), not use the filter (filter always off), or switch the filter on or off by intervening at the time of DXA testing.

The *NOF-ISCD FRAX Implementation Guide* includes a disclaimer of 'This 10 year fracture risk estimate was calculated using FRAX version [X] and a "yes" response for the following FRAX risk factors in this individual: maternal/paternal history of hip fracture, tobacco use, etc.' The *NOF-ISCD Implementation Guide* also provides guidance for determining when a previously treated patient can be considered as untreated for purposes of inclusion in the FRAX tool. Untreated patients include those who, in the past year, have not received estrogen, hormone treatment, a selective estrogen receptor modulator, teriparatide, and denosumab, or, in the past 2 years, a bisphosphonate unless taken orally for less than 2 months. Calcium and vitamin D supplementation are not considered treatment by the *NOF-ISCD FRAX Implementation Guide*.[32,33]

There are important caveats of which DXA center interpreters of BMD and FRAX probabilities and treating clinicians should be aware when using the *NOF-ISCD FRAX Implementation Guide* default filter.[34,35] The default filter does not permit use of FRAX in patients with normal or osteoporotic BMD, although no scientific data exist that substantiate a significant difference in fracture risk between T-scores of −1.0 and −1.1 or between T-scores of −2.4 and −2.5. Healthy younger men and women who have small skeletal structure (small bones) or less than average peak bone mass primarily on a genetic basis without other CRFs for fractures being present may have low FRAX probabilities but are presently being recommended for treatment by the 2008 *NOF Clinician's Guide for the Diagnosis and Treatment of Osteoporosis* (T-score ≤−2.5).[1,36,37] Epidemiologic data do not support treatment of these low-risk patients, and a major nuance of the *Clinician's Guide* compared with previous 2005 NOF guidance supports the premise that fewer young patients at low risk should be treated.[38–40] Patients with normal spine and hip BMD and no prevalent osteoporotic fractures but high FRAX probabilities would not be treated if the default filter was operational. For example, an 85-year-old white woman with specific CRFs (femoral neck T-score of −1.0, smokes, maternal hip fracture, rheumatoid arthritis, corticosteroid treatment) has major osteoporosis and hip fracture probabilities of 39% and 31% respectively, meets the *Clinician's Guide* FRAX high-risk fracture probability thresholds of greater than or equal to 20% for major osteoporosis-related fractures and greater than or equal to 3% for hip fracture for initiation of treatment, but would not have a fracture probability calculated if the default filter was operational. Restricting FRAX to only patients with low bone mass assumes that prospective randomized control trial data are available that confirm the efficacy of pharmacologic treatment in patients with low bone mass but not with normal BMD, a highly controversial subject, whereas recent publications document pharmacologic benefit with or without BMD using FRAX for risk assessment with many, but not all, osteoporosis medications.[39–46] Aligning FRAX to the restrictive randomization criteria used in clinical trials selects patients for treatment based on only clinical trial data and is analogous to the invalid argument of why not to monitor BMD that is primarily derived from similar data.[47] In the National Osteoporosis Risk Assessment (NORA), patients with low-trauma fractures at nonhip and nonvertebral skeletal sites (eg, forearm and ribs) would be filtered out by the default filter with a BMD T-score greater than or equal to −1.0 (normal BMD) and not considered for treatment even though their future fracture risk is high.[48–52] The default filter also excludes patients without an evaluable hip BMD. Although FRAX estimates without inclusion of femoral neck BMD are not as sensitive or predictive of future fracture risk as those inclusive of femoral neck BMD, FRAX without femoral neck BMD can still be useful in providing the clinician and patient with 10-year fracture probabilities that facilitate treatment decisions.[30] Clinicians specializing in osteoporosis frequently use FRAX as part of their initial evaluation of patients who have been prescribed osteoporosis treatment by previous physicians. Although the patient's calculated fracture probabilities are not reliable as a result of being on treatment, it is important for the treating clinician to appreciate, at the time of initial evaluation, a patient's underlying hip and major osteoporosis-related fracture probabilities if they had never been treated with pharmacologic therapy. This additional piece of critical clinical information may be used by the clinician to continue or discontinue therapy or consider a temporary drug holiday. Excluding use of FRAX in these subsets of patients may deprive clinicians and patients' of valuable information not otherwise available.

There are important CRFs that predict future fracture risk but are not incorporated into FRAX and, to variable degrees, in the other available fracture prediction tools, thus limiting each tool's ability to refine a particular risk for the individual patient. An example of a limitation of FRAX is the age range used in the tool, which is between 40 to 90 years. Women who have had a surgical menopause at age 30 years and are not taking hormone treatment would be considered to be 40 years old with the attendant risk of a premenopausal woman. A similar argument has arisen when applying the same rule to a 95 year old who would be classified as being 90 years old. The FRAX CRFs that are treated as dichotomous or yes/no variables can be found in **Table 1**. The inability to adjust the dose and, in many cases, the duration of exposure of the dichotomous CRFs may result in an underestimation or overestimation of hip-related and major osteoporosis-related fracture risk in the patient who is not within the range of CRF dose and duration of use that was initially used for the calculation of risk in the FRAX prospective observational studies.[20,22] Fracture risk associated with the chronic use of high-dose glucocorticoids, exposure to alcohol and tobacco beyond the estimates in the base FRAX populations, a parental history of nonhip fragility fracture, and a personal history of multiple fragility fractures including multiple morphometric vertebral fractures (radiograph confirmed) will all exceed FRAX estimates and thus be underestimated in the calculation of hip-related and major osteoporosis-related 10-year fracture probabilities.

Table 1
FRAX dichotomous clinical risk factors

CRF	Risk Factors
Previous fracture	Spontaneous or low-trauma fracture in adult life (trauma that would not have resulted in fracture in a healthy person)
Parental history of hip fracture	History of hip fracture in patient's mother or father
Current smoking	Presently smoking tobacco
Glucocorticoids (≥3 mo)	Present or past exposure to oral prednisone or its equivalent ≥5 mg/d for more than 3 mo
Rheumatoid arthritis	Confirmed diagnosis of rheumatoid arthritis
Secondary causes	Disease or medical conditions strongly associated with osteoporosis (diabetes mellitus, hypogonadism, premature menopause, osteogenesis imperfecta, untreated hyperthyroidism, malabsorptive diseases, chronic liver disease)
Alcohol	3 or more units per day (1 unit = standard glass of beer, single measure of spirits, medium glass of wine)

Exposure to medications other than prednisone, such as anticonvulsants, lithium, and antiestrogenic and antiandrogenic medications that are known to adversely influence skeletal health are not included in FRAX. Secondary causes that are known to adversely affect skeletal health are only included in the calculation of fracture probability when BMD is not included in the risk calculation. Inclusion of BMD or T-scores into the FRAX tool is limited to the femoral neck because of having the highest gradient of risk of all potential measurement sites for hip fracture. However, it is common that clinicians encounter discordant DXA test results in which the lumbar spine BMD is 1 or more SDs lower than the femoral neck. Nevertheless, inclusion of spine BMD or the equivalent spine T-score instead of femoral neck BMD (or equivalent femoral neck T-score) in the FRAX tool will not generate accurate fracture probabilities for hip-related and major osteoporosis-related fractures.

Up to 30% of seniors living in the community fall each year, with 10% of the falls resulting in hip-related and other major osteoporosis-related fractures and, as such, should be considered in a comprehensive risk management strategy. However, falls are not included in FRAX, other than the assumption that fall risk is included, but are not acknowledged or recorded in the initial cohorts used to construct FRAX.[28,29,53–55] Additional osteoporosis risk calculators are available, including the Garvan Institute fracture risk calculator (Garvan) and QFractureScores (QFracture) fracture prediction tools, which do incorporate falls.[16–19] FRAX does not allow insertion of falls, whereas Garvan provides options for 0, 1, 2, and 3 or more falls in the past 12 months, and QFracture allows a dichotomous yes/no answer for falls within the past 12 months. There are significant differences in the manner in which the 3 calculators were constructed, CRFs entry data, and the definition of osteoporosis fracture probabilities that does not permit a valid comparison between the 3 tools. Despite these differences, it is worthy of note how falls may affect fracture probabilities using FRAX, Garvan, and QFracture, as seen in **Fig. 5**. A summary of the strengths and limitations of FRAX is given in **Table 2**.

FRAX provides the clinician with 10-year hip-related and major osteoporosis-related fracture probabilities but does not provide guidance concerning who should be treated. The 2008 *NOF Clinician's Guide to Prevention and Treatment of Osteoporosis* provides important information about the pathophysiology of osteoporosis, approach to the diagnosis and management of osteoporosis, universal recommendations for all patients, and the pharmacologic and nonpharmacologic management of osteoporosis.[1] The *Clinician's Guide* suggests that pharmacologic treatment decisions be based on high-quality clinical judgment that is inclusive of all available clinical and scientific information and the presence of:

1. Morphometric or clinical vertebral fracture
2. Hip fracture
3. DXA hip (femoral neck) or spine T-score less than or equal to −2.5
4. Low bone mass (osteopenia) and specific WHO FRAX thresholds, adapted to the United States, for hip fracture greater than or equal to 3% or major osteoporosis-related fractures greater than or equal to 20%.

In addition, the *Clinician's Guide* suggests that patient preferences could indicate treatment of people with 10-year fracture probabilities more than or less than these levels.

The *Clinician's Guide* suggested FRAX cut points for initiation of pharmacologic treatment in patients with osteopenia (≥3% for hip fracture and ≥20% for major osteoporosis-related fractures) may not capture specific patients who have sufficient risk to warrant treatment but do not meet the thresholds mentioned earlier because of

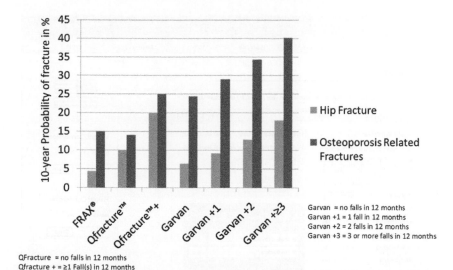

QFracture = no falls in 12 months
Qfracture + = ≥1 Fall(s) in 12 months

Garvan = no falls in 12 months
Garvan +1 = 1 fall in 12 months
Garvan +2 = 2 falls in 12 months
Garvan +3 = 3 or more falls in 12 months

Fig. 5. Falls affect fracture risk. (*Same base patient calculated from*: FRAX, Available at: http://www.shef.ac.uk/FRAX/index.jsp, Garvan Available at: http://www.garvan.org.au/bone-fracture-risk, and QFracture, Available at: http://www.qfracture.org/.)

the dichotomous nature of FRAX CRFs. The potential underestimation of risk using FRAX 3.3 may affect patient selection for pharmacologic intervention according to the *Clinician's Guide* thresholds for pharmacologic intervention, as in the following example. A 65-year-old white patient with a T-score of −1.8 at the femoral neck is prescribed prednisone 60 mg/d for treatment of giant cell arteritis. As seen in **Fig. 6**, the patient's FRAX 10-year hip fracture risk is 2.4% and major osteoporosis-related fracture risk is 15%, which does not meet the *Clinician's Guide* cut point for treatment

Table 2 Strengths and limitations of FRAX	
Strengths of FRAX	**Limitations of FRAX**
1. BMD and easily measured CRFs improve sensitivity of test	Not inclusive of other important CRFs (falls)
2. Dichotomous CRFs	
Previous fracture	Previous multiple fractures, fracture type (hip vs rib), and severity of vertebral fracture(s) are not distinguished
Parental history of hip fracture	Parental nonhip fracture(s) is not included
Current smoking and alcohol	Dose is not included
Glucocorticoids	Dose, duration of use, and other medications that adversely affect bone are not included
Rheumatoid arthritis	RA severity and medications are not included
Secondary causes	Risk is not included if BMD is added to FRAX
3. Femoral neck BMD has highest gradient of risk	Discordantly low spine BMD cannot be used
4. Large population cohorts used to construct FRAX	Single non-FRAX cohort used to independently validate FRAX

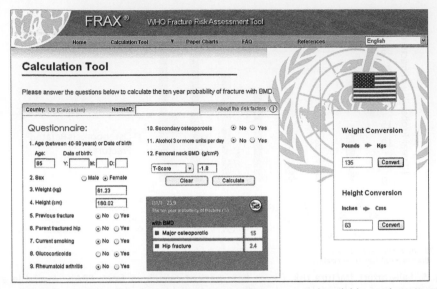

Fig. 6. FRAX with CRF positive for glucocorticoid treatment. (Available at: http://www.sheffield.ac.uk/FRAX/tool.jsp?country59.)

and is inconsistent with the American College of Rheumatology 2010 recommendations for the prevention and treatment of glucocorticoid-induced osteoporosis.[56] The reason for this discrepancy is that FRAX estimates of fracture risk use what is described as an average exposure to prednisone or its equivalent of 2.5 to 7.5 mg/d, which was assumed to be equivalent to the medium dose of glucocorticoid medication used in the UK General Practice Research Database (GPRD).[28,29] In the patient mentioned earlier, FRAX does not take into account higher doses and the potential long-term use of glucocorticoid treatment. Until newer versions of FRAX become available that incorporate population cohorts that allow collection of the variability in CRF exposure, it will be necessary for the physician interpreting bone densitometry tests inclusive of FRAX probabilities and the treating clinician who reviews these results to qualitatively adjust FRAX probabilities according the dose and duration of exposure of individual dichotomous CRFs.

In 2010, the ISCD, in collaboration with the IOF, held a FRAX Position Development Conference (FRAX PDC) that specifically addressed the following topics[28,29]:

- Potential underestimation or overestimation of fracture risk associated with the dichotomous FRAX CRFs
- Clinical usefulness of FRAX without inclusion of BMD
- Integration of the following into FRAX:
  - Other causes of secondary osteoporosis when BMD is also included in FRAX
  - Falls
  - Lumbar spine BMD
  - Biochemical markers of bone turnover
  - Quantitative ultrasound.
- Ethnic and racial variability of FRAX in the United States
- Suggestions for developing FRAX tools internationally.

The joint ISCD and IOF FRAX official positions specifically associated with FRAX CRFs and DXA BMD, described in **Boxes 1–3**, clarified the topics mentioned earlier,

Box 1
Joint ISCD and IOF FRAX official positions

Clinical Risk Factors

1. Impaired functional status in patients with rheumatoid arthritis may be a risk factor for clinical fractures. FRAX may underestimate fracture probability in such patients.

2. There is no consistent evidence that non-glucocorticoid medications for rheumatoid arthritis alter fracture risk.

3. While there is evidence that duration and dose of tobacco smoking may impact on fracture risk, quantification of this risk is not possible.

4. Falls are a risk factor for fractures but are not accommodated as an entry variable in the current FRAX model. Fracture probability may be underestimated in individuals with a history of frequent falls, but quantification of this risk is not currently possible.

5. There is a relationship between number of prior fractures and subsequent fracture risk. FRAX underestimates fracture probability in persons with a history of multiple fractures.

6. There is a relationship between severity of prior vertebral fractures and subsequent fracture risk. FRAX may underestimate fracture probability in individuals with prevalent severe vertebral fractures.

7. While there is evidence that hip, vertebral, and humeral fractures appear to confer greater risk of subsequent fracture than fractures at other sites, quantification of this incremental risk in FRAX is not possible.

Data from Hans D, Kanis J, Baim S, et al. Joint official positions of the International Society for Clinical Densitometry (ISCD) and International Osteoporosis Foundation (IOF) on FRAX: executive Summary of the 2010 Position Development Conference on Interpretation and Use of FRAX® in Clinical Practice. J Clin Densitom 2011. [Epub ahead of print].

Box 2
ISCD and IOF FRAX official positions

Clinical Risk Factors

8. Evidence that bone turnover markers predict fracture risk independent of BMD is inconclusive. Therefore, bone turnover markers are not included as risk factors in FRAX.

9. There is a dose relationship between glucocorticoid use of greater than 3 months and fracture risk. The average dose exposure captured within FRAX is likely to be a prednisone dose of 2.5 to 7.5 mg/d or its equivalent. Fracture probability is under-estimated when prednisone dose is greater than 7.5 mg/d and is over-estimated when prednisone dose is less than 2.5 mg/d.

10. Frequent intermittent use of higher doses of glucocorticoids increases fracture risk. Because of variability in the dose and dosing schedule, quantification of this risk is not possible.

11. High dose inhaled glucocorticoids may be a risk factor for fracture. FRAX may underestimate fracture probability in users of high dose inhaled glucocorticoids.

12. Appropriate glucocorticoid replacement in individuals with adrenal insufficiency has not been shown to increase fracture risk. In such patients, use of glucocorticoids should not be included in FRAX calculations.

Data from Hans D, Kanis J, Baim S, et al. Joint official positions of the International Society for Clinical Densitometry (ISCD) and International Osteoporosis Foundation (IOF) on FRAX: executive Summary of the 2010 Position Development Conference on Interpretation and Use of FRAX® in Clinical Practice. J Clin Densitom 2011. [Epub ahead of print].

Box 3
ISCD and IOF FRAX official positions

Bone Mineral Density

1. Measurements other than BMD or T-score at the femoral neck by DXA are not recommended for use in FRAX.

2. FRAX may underestimate or overestimate major osteoporotic fracture risk when lumbar spine T-score is much lower or higher (>1 SD discrepancy) than femoral neck T-score.

3. A procedure based on the difference (offset) between the LS and FN T-scores can enhance fracture prediction in the current version of FRAX

4. FRAX with BMD predicts fracture risk better than clinical risk factors or BMD alone. Use of FRAX without BMD is appropriate when BMD is not readily available or to identify individuals who may benefit from a BMD measurement.

5. It is not appropriate to use FRAX to monitor treatment response.

6. Evidence that rate of bone loss may be an independent risk factor for fracture is conflicting. Therefore, rate of bone loss is not included as a FRAX risk factor.

Data from Hans D, Kanis J, Baim S, et al. Joint official positions of the International Society for Clinical Densitometry (ISCD) and International Osteoporosis Foundation (IOF) on FRAX: executive Summary of the 2010 Position Development Conference on Interpretation and Use of FRAX in Clinical Practice. J Clin Densitom 2011. [Epub ahead of print].

---

and specifically the base-case inherent risk in the initial cohorts used to construct the dichotomous CRFs, determined whether quantitative or qualitative adjustments to individual CRFs were possible, and provided guidance to those using FRAX about integration of these adjustments into FRAX-generated fracture probabilities.[28,29] The clinical usefulness of qualitative adjustments to hip-related and major osteoporosis-related fracture probability can be appreciated by using the previous example of a 65-year-old white patient with a T-score of −1.8 at the femoral neck who initiated high-dose prednisone 60 mg/d for treatment of giant cell arteritis. The patient's FRAX probabilities are 2.4% and 15% for hip-related and major osteoporosis-related fractures, respectively (see **Fig. 6**). The Joint ISCD and IOF FRAX official position concerning glucocorticoid treatment suggest that this patient's future fracture risk is underestimated because FRAX used a medium dose of prednisone in its base calculation of risk (prednisone 2.5–7.5 mg/d). Hip-related and major osteoporosis-related fracture probabilities should be adjusted higher in this patient to reflect greater risk of fracture. The qualitative adjustment to her major osteoporosis-related fracture risk, as seen in **Fig. 7**, would place this patient in a high-risk category greater than or equal to 20% and, as such, would trigger initiation of treatment according to the *NOF Clinician's Guide* thresholds for treatment intervention. Similar qualitative adjustments to FRAX can now be considered for most dichotomous CRFs by using the guidance offered by the joint ISCD and IOF FRAX official positions.[28,29]

Independent of the joint ISCD and IOF FRAX official positions, additional quantitative adjustments to FRAX hip-related and major osteoporosis-related fracture probabilities using a simplified algorithm are now available for patients treated with prednisone or its equivalent in doses less than 2.5 mg/d (low dose) or greater than 7.5 mg/d (high dose) compared with the base fracture risk used in FRAX (medium dose). **Table 3**[57] describes the simplified algorithm's adjustments to FRAX hip-related and major osteoporosis-related fracture probabilities in accordance with the prescribed glucocorticoid dose. For a patient taking high-dose prednisone (>7.5

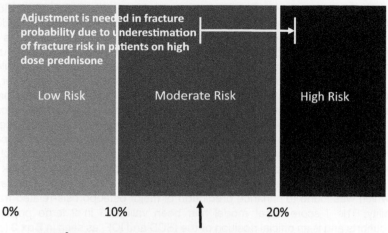

FRAX® calculated10-year major osteoporosis related fracture risk is 15% based on prednisone 2.5-7.5 mg per day in the initial FRAX® population cohort

Fig. 7. Impact of qualitative CRF adjustment in a patient on high-dose prednisone for treatment of giant cell arteritis.

mg/d), FRAX hip-related and major osteoporosis-related fracture probabilities would be increased by 20% and 15%, respectively. Thus, a patient taking high-dose prednisone with a calculated FRAX major osteoporosis-related fracture probability of 18% would have an adjusted probability of 20.7% ($0.18 \times 0.15 + 0.18 \times 100 = 20.7\%$). Some assumptions were made during the development of this simplified algorithm that could potentially limit its accuracy: risk of a major osteoporosis fracture was equivalent to the GPRD for nonvertebral fracture, conservative estimates were made regarding the death hazard because no such data were available in the GPRD, and there is no independent validation of the stated risk estimates as well as correlation with other glucocorticoid-induced fracture incidence data.[57–63]

FRAX probabilities are most accurate when femoral neck BMD is included in the algorithm because of the strength of its association with future hip and other osteoporosis fractures, availability in the FRAX cohorts used to design the algorithm, and is the database used as the reference standard for BMD (NHANES III Caucasian female).[7,64–66] Direct substitution of lumbar spine T-scores into the FRAX algorithm

Table 3		
Adjustments to FRAX for various glucocorticoid doses		
	Adjustments to FRAX	
Prednisone Dose	**Major Fracture**	**Hip Fracture**
Less than 2.5 mg/d	Decrease FRAX probability by 20%	Decrease FRAX probability by 35%
2.5–7.5 mg/d	Stated FRAX estimates	Stated FRAX estimates
Greater than 7.5 mg/d	Increase FRAX probability by 15%	Increase FRAX probability by 20%

Data from Kanis JA, Johansson H, Oden A, et al. Guidance for the adjustment of FRAX according to the dose of glucocorticoids. Osteoporos Int 2011;22:809–16.

results in invalid fracture probabilities because of differences in age-related loss of bone density at different skeletal sites, the frequent occurrence of confounding degenerative changes in the spine (increases measured BMD), significant differences in the gradient of risk between both sites, and the discrepancy in the SD used for calculation of T-scores by DXA manufacturers versus the SD used to determine the gradient of risk in the study populations of the Marshall meta-analysis.[7,67–70] However, it is common for significant discordance of T-scores greater than 1 SD to be present between the femoral neck and lumbar spine regions of interest, resulting in concern about the accuracy of FRAX to predict vertebral fractures.[71] A hybrid model that used lumbar spine BMD to predict spine fractures and femoral neck BMD to predict nonvertebral fractures showed improved sensitivity for spine fracture prediction.[72] This resulted in the development of a simplified model to adjust femoral neck BMD using the difference in T-scores (offset) between the lumbar spine and femoral neck, which was found to enhance prediction of major osteoporosis-related fracture probability. The T-score offset model has been validated in 2 large population-based cohorts and is an official position of the ISCD and IOF, as seen in **Box 3** (official position number 3).[28,73,74] The rule states: "increase/decrease the FRAX estimate for a major osteoporosis-related fracture by one-tenth for each rounded off T-score difference between the lumbar spine and femoral neck."[73,74] Thus a patient with a FRAX major osteoporosis-related fracture risk of 17% who has a femoral neck T-score of −1.5 and a lumbar spine T-score of −3.3 has an offset of −1.8 (−3.3 minus −1.5) or, rounded off, equals 2. The adjusted added risk that takes into account the discordant lower lumbar spine T-score is +3.4% ($0.17 \times 0.1 \times 2 \times 100 = 3.4\%$), which is then added to the base risk of 17% to provide an adjusted major osteoporosis-related fracture risk of 20.4%, as summarized in **Table 4**. Potential adjustments may result in an increase or decrease in major osteoporosis-related fracture probabilities that depends on whether the lumbar spine T-score is less than (worse risk) or greater than (less risk) the femoral neck T-score. All of the calculated adjustments to FRAX probabilities mentioned earlier provide a significant improvement to the prediction of fracture risk in the individual patient.

In summary, using BMD alone to predict low-trauma fractures is associated with low sensitivity that eventuates in greater than 50% of individuals with low-trauma fractures

Table 4
Adjustment to FRAX major osteoporosis-related fracture probability using lumbar spine T-score offset

T-scores	FRAX 10-Year Fracture Probabilities	
	Major Osteoporosis Fractures (%)	Hip Fractures (%)
Before adjustment using femoral neck T-1.5	17.0	2
After adjustment using lumbar spine T-3.3[a]	21.4	2

[a] Calculation of adjustment: T-score offset = −1.8(−3.3 minus −1.5) =>rounded off = 2; adjustment to FRAX = (offset rounded off) × 1/10 × (base fracture risk) × 100 = 2 × 0.10 × 0.17 × 100 = 3.4%; adjusted FRAX major osteoporosis-related fracture risk = 17% + 3.4% = 20.4%.

Data from Leslie WD, Lix LM, Johansson H, et al. Spine-hip discordance and fracture risk assessment: a physician-friendly FRAX enhancement. Osteoporos Int 2011;22:839–47; and Leslie WD, Kovacs CS, Olszynski WP, et al. Spine-Hip T-score difference predicts major osteoporotic fracture risk independent of FRAX®: a population-based report from CAMOS. J Clin Densitom 2011. doi: 10.1016/j.jocd.2011.04.011.

being classified as having osteopenia at the time of initial DXA testing. This concern has resulted in the development of the WHO FRAX fracture prediction algorithm, which combines DXA BMD testing and clinical risk factor assessment to improve fracture prediction. FRAX has been independently validated for prediction of the 10-year fracture probability of hip-related and major osteoporosis-related fractures and is presently being used worldwide as an important component of osteoporosis management strategies for initiation of cost-effective therapies in patients most likely to fracture. It is critical for practicing clinicians and those physicians interpreting DXA BMD with FRAX to appreciate the caveats related to the use of this fracture prediction tool and the various intervention strategies available.

REFERENCES

1. National Osteoporosis Foundation, Clinician's guide to prevention and treatment of osteoporosis. 2008. Available at: http://www.nof.org/professionals/NOF_clinicians_Guide.pdf. Accessed February 12, 2011.
2. Burge R, Dawson-Hughes B, Solomon DH, et al. Incidence and economic burden of osteoporosis-related fractures in the United States, 2005–2025. J Bone Miner Res 2007;3:465–75.
3. World Health Organization (1994) assessment of fracture risk and its application to screening for postmenopausal osteoporosis. Technical report series 843. Geneva (Switzerland): WHO; 1994.
4. Kanis JA, Melton LJ, Christiansen C, et al. The diagnosis of osteoporosis. J Bone Miner Res 1994;9:1137–41.
5. Kanis JA, Johnell O, Oden A, et al. Risk of hip fracture according to the World Health Organization criteria for osteoporosis and osteopenia. Bone 2000;27:585–90.
6. World Health Organization guidelines for preclinical evaluation and clinical trials in osteoporosis. Geneva (Switzerland): WHO; 1998.
7. Marshall D, Johnell O, Edel H. Meta-analysis of how well measures of bone mineral density predict occurrence of osteoporotic fractures. BMJ 1996;312:1254–9.
8. Cooper C, Aihie A. Osteoporosis: recent advances in pathogenesis and treatment. QJM 1994;87:203–9.
9. Kanis JA, Borgstrom F, De Laet C, et al. Assessment of fracture risk. Osteoporos Int 2005;16:581–9.
10. Wainwright SA, Marshall LM, Ensrud KE, et al. Study of Osteoporotic Fractures Research Group. Hip fractures in women without osteoporosis. J Clin Endocrinol Metab 2005;90(5):2787–93.
11. Pasco JA, Seeman E, Henry MJ, et al. The population burden of fractures originates in women with osteopenia, not osteoporosis. Osteoporos Int 2006;17(9): 1404–9.
12. Sornay-Rendu E, Muoz F, Garnero P, et al. Identification of osteopenic women at high risk of fracture. The OFELY study. J Bone Miner Res 2005;20(10):813–1819.
13. Kanis JA, McCloskey EV, Johansson H, et al. Development and use of FRAX® in osteoporosis. Osteoporos Int 2010;21(Suppl 2):S407–13.
14. Papaionnou A, Morin S, Cheung AM, et al. 2010 Clinical practice guidelines for the diagnosis and management of osteoporosis in Canada: summary. CMAJ 2010;182(17):1864–73.
15. Hamdy RC, Baim S, Broy SB. Algorithm for the management of osteoporosis. SMJ 2010;103(10):1009–15.
16. FRAX® Available at: http://www.sheffield.ac.uk/FRAX/index.jsp. Accessed February 24, 2011.

17. World Health Organization. Assessment of osteoporosis at the primary health care level. WHO, Geneva (Switzerland), 2007. Available at: www.who.int/chp/topics/rheumatic/en/index.html. Accessed February 23, 2011.
18. Nguyen ND, Frost SA, Center JR, et al. Development of prognostic nomograms for individualizing 5-year and 10-year fracture risks. Osteoporos Int 2008;19: 1431–44. Available at: http://www.garvan.org.au/bone-fracture-risk. Accessed February 24, 2011.
19. Hippisley-Cox J, Copuland C. Predicting risk of osteoporotic fracture in men and women in England and Wales: prospective derivation and validation of QFractureScores. BMJ 2009;339:b4229. Available at: http://www.qfracture.org/. Accessed February 24, 2011.
20. Kanis JA on behalf of the World Health Organization Scientific Group a, Assessment of osteoporosis at the primary health-care level. Technical Report. WHO Collaborating Centre, University of Sheffield. UK; 2008. Available at: http://www.shef.ac.uk/FRAX/index.htm. Accessed February 24, 2011.
21. Oden A, Johansson H, McCloskey EV. FRAX™ and the assessment of fracture probability in men and women from the UK. Osteoporos Int 2008;19:385–97.
22. Kanis JA, Johnell O, Oden A, et al. FRAX and the assessment of fracture probability in men and women from the UK. Osteoporos Int 2008;19:385–97.
23. FRAX. Available at: http://www.shef.ac.uk//FRAX. Accessed February 23, 2011.
24. Kanis JA, Oden A, Johnell O, et al. The use of clinical risk factors enhances the performance of BMD in the prediction of hip and osteoporotic fractures in men and women. Osteoporos Int 2007;18:1033–46.
25. Schousboe JT, Vokes T, Broy SB, et al. Vertebral fracture assessment, The 2007 Official Positions. JCD 2008;11:92–108.
26. Available at: http://itunes.apple.com/us/app/frax/id370146412?mt=8. Accessed February 24, 2011.
27. Available at: http://www.shef.ac.uk/FRAX/charts.jsp. Accessed February 24, 2011.
28. Hans D, Kanis J, Baim S, et al. Joint official positions of the International Society for Clinical Densitometry (ISCD) and International Osteoporosis Foundation (IOF) on FRAX®: executive Summary of the 2010 Position Development Conference on Interpretation and Use of FRAX® in Clinical Practice. J Clin Densitom 2011. [Epub ahead of print].
29. Kanis J, Hans D, Cooper C, et al. Interpretation and use of FRAX® in clinical practice. Osteoporos Int 2011. Epub.
30. Leslie WD, Lix LM, Johansson H, et al. Independent clinical validation of a Canadian FRAX tool: fracture prediction and model calibration. J Bone Miner Res 2010;25(11):2350–8.
31. Fraser L-A, Langsetmo L, Berger C, et al. Fracture prediction and calibration of a Canadian FRAX tool: a population-based report from CaMos. Osteoporos Int 2011;22:829–37.
32. FRAX implementation guide. Available at: http://www.nof.org/sites/default/files/pdfs/nof_FRAX_Implem_Guide.pdf. Accessed February 24, 2011.
33. FRAX implementation guide. Available at: http://www.iscd.org/visitors/pdfs/FRAXimplementationGuide_000.pfd. Accessed February 24, 2011.
34. Watts NB, Siris ES, Cummings SR, et al. Perspective: filtering FRAX®. Osteoporos Int 2010;21:537–41.
35. McCloskey E, Compston J, Cooper C. The US FRAX® filter: avoiding confusion or hindering progress? Osteoporos Int 2010;21:885.
36. Tosteson AN, Melton LJ, Dawson-Hughes B, et al. Cost-effective osteoporosis treatment thresholds: the United States perspective. Osteoporos Int 2008;19:437–47.

37. Dawson-Hughes B, Tostoson ANA, Melton LJ, et al. Implications of absolute fracture risk assessment for osteoporosis practice guidelines in the USA. Osteoporos Int 2008;19:449–58.
38. Leslie WD, Tsang JF, Lix LM. Effect of total hip bone area on osteoporosis diagnosis and fractures. J Bone Miner Res 2008;23:1468–76.
39. Dawson-Hughes B, Looker AC, Tosteson ANA, et al. The potential impact of new National Osteoporosis Foundation guidance on treatment patterns. Osteoporos Int 2010;21:41–52.
40. Cummings SR, Ensrud K, Donaldson MG, et al. The US National Osteoporosis Foundation (NOF) Guidelines: recommendations for pharmacologic treatment. IBMS Bone Key 2008;5:137–41.
41. Cauley JA, Robbins J, Chen Z, et al. Effects of estrogen plus progestin on risk of fracture and bone mineral density: the Women's Health Initiative randomized trial. JAMA 2003;290:1729–38.
42. Kanis JA, Oden A, Johansson H, et al. FRAX® and its applications to clinical practice. Bone 2009;44:734–43.
43. McCloskey EV, Johansson H, Oden A, et al. Ten-year fracture probability identifies women who benefit from clodronate therapy-additional results from a double-blind, placebo-controlled randomized study. Osteoporos Int 2009;20:811–7.
44. Kanis JA, Johansson H, Oden A, et al. Bazedoxifene reduces vertebral and clinical fractures in postmenopausal women at high risk assessed with FRAX. Bone 2009;44:1049–54.
45. Kanis JA, Johansson H, Oden A, et al. A meta-analysis of the efficacy of raloxifene on all clinical and vertebral fractures and its dependency on FRAX®. Bone 2010;47:729–35.
46. Kanis JA, Johansson H, Oden A. A meta-analysis of the effect of strontium ranelate on the risk of vertebral and non-vertebral fracture in postmenopausal osteoporosis and the interaction with FRAX®. Osteoporos Int 2011;22(8):2347–55.
47. Watts NB, Lewiecki EM, Bonnick SL, et al. Clinical value of monitoring BMD in patients treated with bisphosphonates for osteoporosis. J Bone Miner Res 2009;24:1643–6.
48. Barrett-Conner E, Sajjan SG, Siris ES, et al. Wrist fracture as a predictor of future fractures in younger versus older postmenopausal women: results from the National Osteoporosis Risk Assessment (NORA). Osteoporos Int 2008;19:607–13.
49. Siris ES, Chen YT, Abbott TA, et al. Bone mineral density threshold for pharmacologic intervention to prevent fractures. Obstet Gynecol Surv 2004;59(1):769–71.
50. Barrett-Connor E, Sajjan SG, Miller PD, et al. Rib fracture as an indicator of future fracture risk in postmenopausal women 50–99 years of age: results from the National Osteoporosis Risk Assessment (NORA). Osteoporos Int 2006;17:S145.
51. Ismail AA, Silman AJ, Reeve J, et al. Rib fractures predict incident limb fractures: results from the European prospective osteoporosis study. Osteoporos Int 2006; 17:41–5.
52. Palvanen M, Kannus P, Niemi S, et al. Hospital-treated minimal-trauma rib fractures in elderly Finns: long-term trend and projections for the future. Osteoporos Int 2004;15:649–53.
53. Gillespie LD, Robertson MC, Lamb SE, et al. 2010 Interventions for preventing falls in older people living in the community (review); The Cochrane Collaboration. Available at: http://onlinelibrary.wiley.com/o/cochrane/clsysrev/articles/CD007146/frame.html. Accessed February 24, 2011.
54. Cameron ID, Murray GR, Gillespie LD, et al. 2010 Interventions for preventing falls in older people in nursing care facilities and hospitals (review). Available

at: http://onlinelibrary.wiley.com/o/cochrane/clsysrev/articles/CD005465/frame.html. Accessed February 25, 2011.

55. Howe TE, Rochester L, Jackson A, 2008 exercise for improving balance in older people (review). Available at: http://onlinelibrary.wiley.com/o/cochrane/clsysrev/articles/CD004963/frame.html. Accessed February 25, 2011.

56. Grossman JM, Gordon R, Ranganath VK, et al. American College of Rheumatology 2010 recommendations for the prevention and treatment of glucocorticoid-induced osteoporosis. Arthritis Care Res 2010;62(11):1515–26.

57. Kanis JA, Johansson H, Oden A, et al. Guidance for the adjustment of FRAX according to the dose of glucocorticoids. Osteoporos Int 2011;22:809–16.

58. Kanis article above van Staa TP, Leufkens HG, Abenhaim L, et al. Oral corticosteroids and fracture risk: relationship to daily and cumulative doses. Rheumatology(Oxford) 2000;39:1383–9.

59. Reid DM, Hughes RA, Laan RF, et al. Efficacy and safety of daily risedronate in the treatment of corticosteroid-induced osteoporosis in men and women: a randomized trial. J Bone Miner Res 2000;15(6):1006–13.

60. Michel BA, Bloch DA, Wolfe F, et al. Fractures in rheumatoid arthritis: an evaluation of associated risk factors. J Rheumatol 1993;20(10):1666–9.

61. Reid IR. Glucocorticoid osteoporosis-mechanisms and management. Eur J Endocrinol 1997;137:209–17.

62. Cooper C, Coupland C, Mitchell M. Rheumatoid arthritis, corticosteroid therapy and hip fracture. Ann Rheum Dis 1995;54:49–52.

63. De Vries F, Brache M, Leufkens HG, et al. Fracture risk with intermittent high-dose oral glucocorticoid therapy. Arthritis Rheum 2007;56:208–14.

64. Johnell O, Kanis JA, Oden A, et al. Predictive value of BMD for hip and other fractures. J Bone Miner Res 2005;20:1185–94.

65. Kanis JA, McCloskey EV, Johansson H, et al. A reference standard for the description of osteoporosis. Bone 2008;42:467–75.

66. Looker AC, Wahner HW, Dunn WL, et al. Updated data on proximal femur bone mineral levels of US adults. Osteoporos Int 1998;8:468–89.

67. Jones G, Nguyen T, Sambrook PN, et al. A longitudinal study of the effect of spinal degenerative disease on bone density in the elderly. J Rheumatol 1995; 22:932–6.

68. Phillipov G, Phillips PJ. Skeletal site bone mineral density heterogeneity in women and men. Osteoporos Int 2001;12:362–5.

69. Schneider DL, Bettencourt R, Barrett-Connor E. Clinical utility of spine bone density in elderly women. J Clin Densitom 2006;9:255–60.

70. Faulkner KG, von Stetten E, Miller P. Discordance in patient classification using T-scores. J Clin Densitom 1999;2:343–50.

71. Leslie WD, Lix LM, Tsang JF, et al. Single-site vs multisite bone density measurement for fracture prediction. Arch Intern Med 2007;167:1641–7.

72. Leslie WD, Lix LM. Absolute fracture risk assessment using lumbar spine and femoral neck bone density measurements: derivation and validation of a hybrid system. J Bone Miner Res 2011;26:460–7.

73. Leslie WD, Lix LM, Johansson H, et al. Spine-hip discordance and fracture risk assessment: a physician-friendly FRAX enhancement. Osteoporos Int 2011;22:839–47.

74. Leslie WD, Kovacs CS, Olszynski WP, et al. Spine-hip T-score difference predicts major osteoporotic fracture risk independent of FRAX®: a population-based report from CAMOS. J Clin Densitom 2011;11(1):123–62.

Teriparitide Update

Stuart L. Silverman, MD[a,b,c,]*, Keaton Nasser, MD[b]

KEYWORDS

- Teriparitide • Osteoporosis • Postmenopausal women
- Osteonecrosis

In postmenopausal osteoporotic women, the benefits of both bisphosphonates and teriparatide (TPD) in reducing fracture risk are well established. Unlike bisphosphonates, which reduce bone resorption, TPD is an anabolic agent that stimulates bone formation initially, then stimulates bone turnover with bone formation exceeding bone resorption.

TPD was found in a pivotal fracture trial to reduce risk of radiographic vertebral fracture by 70%, clinical vertebral fracture by 77% and nonvertebral fracture by 68%.[1] TPD was approved for daily self-injection for up to 2 years. The availability of an anabolic agent that could improve microarchitecture has opened up a new paradigm in osteoporosis treatment. However, many questions still remain:

Can gains be maximized by combining with an antiresorptive therapy?
What should follow a course of TPD therapy?
Is daily therapy the only option, or can one consider cyclic therapy?
How well do patients with prior antiresorptive therapy respond to TPD?
Does TPD have other indications than postmenopausal osteoporosis?
Does TPD reduce pain in patients with osteoporosis?

COMBINATION TREATMENT WITH TPD AND ZOLEDRONIC ACID

TPD increases bone formation initially within the first month but then increases bone turnover with formation exceeding resorption. It is therefore of interest to see if combination therapy with a potent bisphosphonate would allow bone formation to continue unheeded. Earlier work in the Parathyroid Hormone and Alendronate for Osteoporosis trial by Black[2] showed that concomitant treatment with an oral bisphosphonate reduced the bone mineral density (BMD) response to parathyroid hormone, with a twofold increase in volumetric BMD with TPD alone compared with TPD and

---

[a] Cedars-Sinai Bone Center of Excellence, 8641 Wilshire Boulevard, Suite 301, Beverly Hills, CA 90211, USA
[b] OMC Clinical Research Center, Beverly Hills, CA, USA
[c] David Geffen School of Medicine, University of California Los Angeles, Los Angeles, CA, USA
* Corresponding author. Cedars-Sinai Bone Center of Excellence, 8641 Wilshire Boulevard, Suite 301, Beverly Hills, CA 90211.
E-mail address: stuarts@omcresearch.org

Rheum Dis Clin N Am 37 (2011) 471–477
doi:10.1016/j.rdc.2011.08.002
0889-857X/11/$ – see front matter © 2011 Published by Elsevier Inc.

alendronate. There was no evidence for synergy. However, animal studies showed that this response reduction did not occur with a parenteral bisphosphonate. Cosman and colleagues[3] recently evaluated the effects of combination therapy with an infusion of a parenteral bisphosphonate, zoledronic acid 5 mg and daily TPD for 1 year. Four hundred twelve postmenopausal women were randomized to a single infusion of zoledronic acid plus TPD (n = 137), zoledronic acid alone (n = 137), or teriparatide alone (n = 138). Bone markers and BMD were measured. After 1 year, lumbar spine BMD had increased 7.5%, 7.0%, and 4.4% in the combination, TPD, and zoledronic acid groups, respectively (P>.001). In the combination group, spine BMD increased more rapidly than with either agent alone (P<.001 at 13 and 26 weeks). Combination therapy increased total-hip BMD more than TPD alone at all times (all P<.01) and more than zoledronic acid at 13 weeks, with final 52-week increments of 2.3%, 1.1%, and 2.2% in the combination, TPD, and zoledronic acid groups. With combination therapy, a marker of bone formation procollagen type 1 amino terminal propeptide increased with levels above baseline from 6 to 12 months. A marker of Bone resorption C-telopeptide was markedly reduced with combination therapy from 0 to 8 weeks (a reduction of similar magnitude to that seen with zoledronic acid alone), followed by a gradual increase with levels remaining above baseline for the remainder of the study. Levels for both markers were significantly lower with combination therapy versus TPD alone. The results did not show a distinct advantage at 1 year for combination therapy but did show earlier BMD increases at the hip.

PRIOR BISPHOSPHONATE TREATMENT

An earlier study by Ettinger[4] studied patients previously treated with alendronate or raloxifene. Alendronate prevented BMD increases in the first 6 months, which raloxifene did not. In European Study of Forsteo (EUROFORS),[5] a European observational study of TPD, this delay was not observed in patients previously treated with alendronate, etidronate, or risedronate. One explanation may be the compliance of the patients on alendronate. In the Ettinger study, the patients were all chosen to have been at least 80% compliant, while this was not a criterion in EUROFORS.

FOLLOW-UP TREATMENT

The approval of TPD by the US Food and Drug Administration (FDA) was issued with the recommendation that treatment last no longer than 2 years. However, there were no recommendations about treatment options thereafter. Studies suggest gains achieved in BMD are lost if an antiresorptive agent is not administered after treatment. Black and colleagues[6] examined the effect of alendronate compared with placebo therapy after at least 1 year of parathyroid hormone (PTH) (1–84). Over 2 years, alendronate therapy after PTH (1–84) led to significant increases in BMD compared with placebo. After 1 year of PTH (1–84), BMD gains appear to be maintained or increased with alendronate, but lost if treatment is not followed by an antiresorptive agent. The use of a potent antiresorptive agent after treatment with TPD thus creates a second anabolic window. Rittmaster[7] found enhancement of the BMD gains after discontinuation of TPD and institution of alendronate therapy, with a 7.1% gain in lumbar spine BMD after 1 year and a 13.4% gain after TPD and 1 year alendronate. The declines in BMD after stopping TPD appear greater in women than men.[8] One of the authors (SLS) of this article currently uses either parenteral bisphosphonate or denosumab after completion of a course of TPD.

A related question is whether patients who have been treated with TPD will benefit from retreatment. Finkelstein[9] reported that patients treated with TPD had a 12.5%

increase in lumbar spine BMD after 1 year. After a 1 year hiatus, the patients responded again but to a lesser extent to TPD (BMD gains in lumbar spine of 5.2%).

CYCLIC TPD

TPD stimulates bone formation within 1 month. Indexes of bone remodeling then peak and plateau, with bone formation exceeding bone resorption, but then slowly decline. The cause of this resistance to continued treatment is unknown but may be associated with increasing serum levels of DKK1, a specific Wnt antagonist,[10] and resulted in a 2-year treatment window for TPD. Cosman and colleagues[11] evaluated whether, for women on concomitant alendronate therapy, short, 3-month cycles of teriparatide could be effective as continuous daily administration. In both groups, bone formation indexes increased quickly. For women receiving cycling therapy, bone formation declined during cycles without TPD. Bone resorption increased in both groups, but increased progressively more in the daily treatment group. Spine BMD increased 6.1% in the daily treatment group and 5.4% in the cyclic group. This study suggests that in patients with osteoporosis after prior alendronate treatment, both daily and cyclic treatment regimens may increase BMD. The effect of cyclic regimens on fracture efficacy is, however, not known.

FRACTURE HEALING WITH TPD

In osteoporosis, TPD is used as an anabolic agent to stimulate bone formation by enhancing osteoblast-derived bone formation to increase bone mass. Fracture healing follows a similar path, requiring increased bone formation at the fracture site for repair.[12] Research is underway to determine the effects of TPD on mesenchymal stem cells to aide in fracture healing.[7]

Basic science research in rat and monkey models shows promising results in the use of TPD for fracture healing. Andreassen and colleagues[13,14] showed that doses of 60 to 200 μg/kg (considerably more than the human dose) caused a more mature callus to form more rapidly than the control group. Alkhiary and colleagues[15] used even lower doses, 5 to 30 μg/kg, in a rat model that showed marked increases in volume, stiffness, torsional strength, and BMD of the callus. Other rat and mice model studies have shown similar results.[16-18] O'Loughlin and colleagues[19] looked at the influence of TPD in rabbit spine fusion. With 10 μg/kg, fusion rate improved 30% to 81%, and histology showed a twofold increased in bone area and a tenfold increase in cartilage formation. Manabe and colleagues[20] demonstrated that TPD accelerated fracture healing in a larger study in a femoral osteotomy model in cynomologous monkeys.

There have been anecdotal and case report studies with TPD improving healing in people.[21-23] However, there has been only 1 randomized, double-blind, controlled trial studying TPD for accelerated fracture healing, which showed only mixed results. One hundred two postmenopausal women with distal radius fracture were randomized to receive daily injections of placebo, 20 μg of TPD, or 40 μg of TPD for 8 weeks. Therapy was initiated within 10 days of fracture. Radiographs were taken every 2 weeks. In comparing the time to bridging of 3 of 4 cortices, there was no significant difference between the placebo group and 40 μg group (median time 9.1 and 8.8 weeks, respectively). Median time to bridging for the 20 μg group was statistically different at 7.4 weeks ($P = .006$); however, due to differences in the calculation of the 95% confidence interval (CI) for the 20 μg and 40 μg TPD groups, comparisons of median time to healing between the 2 TPD groups were not significantly different. Median time to bridging of 4 cortices was similar between all groups (11.3 weeks, 10.9 weeks, and 11.0 weeks for placebo, 20 μg, and 40 μg treatment groups, respectively), and there were no statistical differences in grip strength or reported pain between the 3 groups.[24] The trial did not look at an early marker of bone healing, callus formation. Aspenberg[25] examined callus formation at 5 weeks in a subset of the patients enrolled at his hospital. TPD appeared to improve early callus formation.

HEALING OF ATYPICAL FEMORAL FRACTURES

Based on the reports of fracture healing of stress fractures in rodents, there have been anecdotal reports of healing of bilateral subtrochanteric fractures in women exposed to long-term bisphosphonate therapy.[26,27]

USE IN OSTEONECROSIS OF THE JAW AND OSSEOUS INTEGRATION OF TITANIUM JAW IMPLANTS

Based on TPD's known anabolic effect and its presumed role in accelerating bone healing, there have been case reports of healing of bisphosphonate-associated osteonecrosis of the jaw.[28]

TPD has also been studied with regards to osseointegration of titanium dental implants where greater new bone volume was seen with TPD versus placebo.[29] TPD compared with placebo also had greater resolution of alveolar bone deficits and accelerated osseous wound healing in patients with severe,chronic peridontitis undergoing periodontal surgery.[30]

USE IN RENAL DISEASE

Adynamic bone disease (ABD) in chronic renal failure patients on dialysis is defined as a very low bone turnover state associated with functional hypoparathyroidism. The use of an anabolic agent such as teriparatide would be a plausible approach to management of ABD. A pilot study by Cejka in 7 patients with ABD showed significant increases in lumbar spine BMD without significant changes in bone turnover markers.[31] Further clinical studies are needed.

USE IN TRANSIENT OSTEOPOROSIS OF THE HIP

Transient osteoporosis may present clinically as several-month history of increasing pain with abnormal magnetic resonance imaging (MRI) scans but normal radiographs. A case report noted disappearance of symptoms and normalization of MRI findings with a 1-month course of TPD[32]; however, this is a condition that may disappear and normalize on its own. No conclusions can therefore be drawn.

REDUCTION IN PAIN

TPD has been anecdotally reported to decrease pain in osteoporosis. An observational study of teriparatide use in Europe in postmenopausal women who received TPD for at least 12 months found significant reductions in back pain regardless of the presence of recent vertebral fracture.[33]

However, a randomized controlled trial comparing risedronate with TPD in patients with back pain thought to be due to osteoporosis showed no treatment effect.[34]

ROLE OF TPD IN THE TREATMENT OF GLUCOCORTICOID-INDUCED OSTEOPOROSIS

One of the most important adverse effects of glucocorticoids is bone loss and the development of glucocorticoid-induced osteoporosis (GIOP), which leads to increased risk of fracture.

Bone loss with glucorticoids occurs through multiple mechanisms. There is an early rapid phase of bone resorption in the first year followed by long-term effects on osteoblast numbers and function. Glucocorticoids decrease osteoblastogenesis and increase apoptosis of both osteoblasts and osteocytes.[35]

Since TPD has a predominant anabolic effect on bone, it has been considered a treatment option since the first study by Lane in 1998, which showed dramatic increases in lumbar spine BMD and quantitative computerized tomography in patients treated with TPD versus those treated with estrogen therapy only.[36]

Saag and colleagues[37] conducted a randomized controlled trial comparing TPD with alendronate. After 36 months of follow-up, there was a significantly greater increase in lumbar spine BMD in the TPD group at 11% compared with 5.3% gain in the alendronate group ($P<.001$). Greater increases were also seen with teriparatide at hip sites. Although fracture was not the primary endpoint, there were less fractures in the TPD arm, with 1.7% (3/173) of patients on TPD found to have a new vertebral fracture compared with 7.7% (13 of 169 patients) in the alendronate group. TPD is an efficacious agent in the treatment of GIOP and may play an important role in the management of patients with GIOP with fracture.

ADHERENCE TO TERIPARATIDE

The authors recognize that adherence to oral osteoporosis medications is low. TPD requires daily self-injection for up to 2 years and may have significant out-of-pocket costs for some patients. Foster and colleagues studied compliance and persistence to TPD in a medical claims database.[38] The results showed adherence better than published data with oral bisphosphonates. Persistence of TPD was 64.6% at 6 months and 56.7% at 12 months. Lower copays were associated with greater persistence, as was prior use of an antiresorptive.

SUMMARY

TPD is a novel anabolic agent that has changed the paradigms of osteoporosis and metabolic bone disease treatment by its mechanism of action of enhancing bone formation.

TPD has been shown to be effective in reducing fracture risk in postmenopausal osteoporosis and has shown significant BMD increases in GIOP with a secondary effect on vertebral fracture reduction greater than a bisphosphonate. Further studies are needed to better understand how to optimize use of this novel agent and to explore other potential uses.

REFERENCES

1. Neer RM, Arnauld CD, Zanchetta JR, et al. Effect of PTH 1,34 on fracture and BMD in postmenopausal women with osteoporosis. N Engl J Med 2001;344: 1434–41.
2. Black DM, Greenspan SL, Ensrud KE, et al. The effects of parathyroid hormone and alendronate alone or in combination in postmenopausal osteoporosis. N Engl J Med 2003;349:1207–15.
3. Cosman F, Eriksen EF, Recknor C, et al. Effects of intravenous zoledronic acid plus subcutaneous teriparatide [rhPTH(1–34)] in postmenopausal osteoporosis. J Bone Miner Res 2011;26:503–11.
4. Ettinger B, San Martin J, Crans G, et al. Differential effects of teriparatide on BMD after treatment with raloxifene or alendronate. J Bone Miner Res 2004;19:745–51.

5. Boonen S, Marin F, Obermayer-Pietsch B, et al. Effects of previous antiresorptive therapy on BMD response to two years teriparatide therapy in postmenopausal women with osteoporosis. J Clin Endocrinol Metab 2008;93:852–60.

6. Black DM, Bilezikian JP, Ensrud KE. One year of alendronate after one year of parathyroid hormone (1–84) for osteoporosis. N Engl J Med 2005;353:555–65.

7. Rittmaster RS, Bolognese M, Ettinger MP, et al. Enhancement of bone mass in osteoporotic women with PTH followed by alendronate. J Clin Endocrinol Metab 2000;85:2129–34.

8. Leder BZ, Neer RM, Wyland JJ, et al. Effects of teriparatide treatment and discontinuation in postmenopausal women and eugonadal men with osteoporosis. J Clin Endocrinol Metab 2009;94:2915–21.

9. Finkelstein JS, Wyland JJ, Leder BZ, et al. Effects of teriparatide retreatment in osteoporotic men and women. J Clin Endocrinol Metab 2009;94:2495–501.

10. Gatti D, Viapiana O, Idolazzi L, et al. The waning of teriparatide effect on bone formation markers in postmenopausal osteoporosis is associated with increasing serum levels of DKK1. J Clin Endocrinol Metab 2011;96:1555–9.

11. Cosman F, Nieves J, Zion M, et al. Daily and cyclic parathyroid hormone in women receiving alendronate. N Engl J Med 2005;353:566–75.

12. Bukata SV, Puzas JE. Orthopedic uses of teriparatide. Curr Osteoporos Rep 2010;8:28–33.

13. Andreassen TT, Ejersted C, Oxlund H. Intermittent parathyroid hormone (1–34) treatment increases callus formation and mechanical strength of healing rat fractures. J Bone Miner Res 1999;14:960–8.

14. Andreassen TT, Willick GE, Morley P, et al. Treatment with parathyroid hormone hPTH(1–34), hPTH(1–31), and monocyclic hPTH(1–31) enhances fracture strength and callus amount after withdrawal fracture strength and callus mechanical quality continue to increase. Calcif Tissue Int 2004;74:351–6.

15. Alkhiary YM, Gerstenfeld LC, Krall E, et al. Enhancement of experimental fracture healing by systemic administration of recombinant human parathyroid hormone (PTH 1–34). J Bone Joint Surg Am 2005;87:731–41.

16. Friedl G, Turner RT, Evans GL, et al. Intermittent parathyroid hormone (PTH) treatment and age-dependent effects on rat cancellous bone and mineral metabolism. J Orthop Res 2007;25:1454–64.

17. Nakazawa T, Nakajima A, Shiomi K, et al. Effects of low-dose, intermittent treatment with recombinant human parathyroid hormone (1–34) on chondrogenesis in a model of experimental fracture healing. Bone 2005;37:711–9.

18. Kakar S, Einhorn TA, Vora S, et al. Enhanced chondrogenesis and Wnt signaling in PTH-treated fractures. J Bone Miner Res 2007;22:1903–12.

19. O'Loughlin PF, Cunningham ME, Bukata SV, et al. Parathyroid hormone (1–34) augments spinal fusion, fusion mass volume, and fusion mass quality in a rabbit spinal fusion model. Spine (Phila Pa 1976) 2009;34:121–30.

20. Manabe T, Mori S, Mashiba T, et al. Human parathyroid hormone (1–34) accelerates natural fracture healing process in the femoral osteotomy model of cynomolgus monkeys. Bone 2007;40:1475–82.

21. Resmini G, Iolascon G. 79-year-old postmenopausal woman with humerus fracture during teriparatide treatment. Aging Clin Exp Res 2007;19:30–1.

22. Peichl P, Krankenhaus Wien Waehring E, Holzer G. Parathyroid hormone (1–84) accelerates fracture healing in pubic bones of elderly osteoporotic women. J Bone Miner Res 2009;24(Suppl 1). Available at: http://www.asbmr.org/Meetings/AnnualMeetings/AbstractDetail.aspx?aid=9d4e83f0-6302-4327-8a9d-758dc56cc703. Accessed August 20, 2011.

23. Bukata SV, Kaback L, Reynolds D, et al. 1–34 PTH at physiological doses in humans shows promise as a helpful adjuvant in difficult to heal fractures: an observational cohort of 145 patients. Presented at the 55th Annual Meeting of the Orthopaedic Research Society. Las Vegas (Nevada), February 25, 2009.

24. Aspenberg P, Genant HK, Johansson T. Teriparatide for accelaration of fracture repair in humans: a prospective randomized double blind study of 102 postmenopausal women with distal radial fractures. J Bone Miner Res 2010;25: 404–14.

25. Aspenberg P, Johansson T. Teriparatide improves early callus formation in distal radial fractures. Acta Orthop 2010;81:234–6.

26. Gomberg SJ, Wustrack RL, Napoli N, et al. Teriparatide, vitamin D and calcium-healed bilateral subtrochanteric stress fractures in a postmenopausal woman with a 13-year history of continuous alendronate therapy. J Clin Endocrinol Metab 2011;96:1627–32.

27. Carvalho NN, Voss LA, Almeida MO, et al. Atypical fremoral fractures during prolonged use of bisphosphonates: short term responses to strontium ranelate and teriparatide. J Clin Endocrinol Metab 2011. [Epub ahead of print].

28. Narongroeknawin P, Danila M, Humphreys LG Jr, et al. Bisphosphonate associated 27. osteonecrosis of the jaw, with healing after teriparatide: a review of the literature and a case report. Spec Care Dentist 2010;30:77–82.

29. Kuchler U, Luvizuto ER, Tangl S, et al. Short term teriparatide delivery and osseointegration: a clinical feasibility study. J Dent Res 2011;90:1001–6.

30. Bashutski JD, Eber RM, Kinney JS, et al. Teriparatide and osseous regeneration in the oral cavity. N Engl J Med 2010;363:2396–405.

31. Cejka D, Kodras K, Bader T, et al. Treatment of hemodialysis associated adynamic bone disease with teriparatide: a pilot study. Kidney Blood Press Res 2010;33:221–6.

32. Fabbriciani G, Pirro M, Manfredelli M, et al. Transient osteoporosis of the hip: successful treatment with teriparatide. Rheumatol Int 2010. [Epub ahead of print].

33. Lyritis G, Marin F, Barker C, et al. Back pain during different sequential treatment regimens of teriparitide: results from Eurofors. Curr Med Res Opin 2010;26: 1799–807.

34. Petal H. Effect of teriparatide compared with risedonate on back pain and incident vertebral fractures in postmenopausal women with ostropeodic vertebral fractures Presented at European Calcified Tissue Society. May 7–11, Athenes, Greece, 2011.

35. Canalis E, Bilezikian JP, Angeli A, et al. Perspectives on glucocorticoid induced osteoporosis. Bone 2004;34:593–8.

36. Love NE, Sanchez S, Modin GW. Parathyroid hormone treatment can reverse corticosteroid-induced osteoporosis: results of a randomized controlled clinical trial. J Clin Invest 1998;102:1627–33.

37. Saag KG, Zanchetta JR, Devogelaer JP, et al. Effects of teriparatide versus alendronate for treating glucocorticoid-induced osteoporosis: thirty-six months results of a randomized, double-blind, controlled trial. Arthritis Rheum 2009;60: 3346–55.

38. Foster SA, Foley KA, Meadows ES, et al. Adherence and persistence with teriparatide among patients with commercial, Medicare, and Medicaid insurance. Osteoporos Int 2011;22:551–7.

Index

Note: Page numbers of article titles are in **boldface** type.

A

Acid phosphatase, tartrate-resistant, assays for, 371
Alendronate
  complications from, 381
  discontinuation of
    bone mineral density effects of, 324–325
    bone turnover marker effects of, 324–325
    fracture risk after, 327–332
  esophageal cancer due to, 394–395
  for glucocorticoid-induced osteoporosis, 419–421
  for men, 407
  response to, bone turnover markers for, 377–378
  selection of, bone turnover markers for, 374–375
  teriparatide after, 474
  transitioning to denosumab, 445
  versus denosumab, 445–447
Alendronate Phase III Treatment Group, 324–325, 327–328
Alkaline phosphatase, bone-specific. *See* BSAP (bone-specific alkaline phosphatase).
American Academy of Oral and Maxillofacial Surgeons, osteonecrosis of jaw
  definition of, 388–389
American College of Physicians, osteoporosis screening guidelines of, 404
American College of Rheumatologists, recommendations, 422–427
American Society for Bone and Mineral Research task force, osteonecrosis of jaw
  definition of, 389
Amino-terminal crosslinking telopeptide of type I collagen. *See* NTX
  (amino-terminal crosslinking telopeptide of type I collagen).
Anabolic agents, 342–348
Androgen deprivation therapy
  denosumab with, 447
  osteoporosis in, 403–404
Antiresorptive agents. *See also specific agents, eg.* Bisphosphonates.
  complications of, **387–400**
  new, 339–342
  safety of, **387–400**
Aromatase inhibitors, denosumab with, 447–448
Atherosclerosis, vitamin D and calcium supplementation and, 356–357
Autoimmune disease, vitamin D and, 358–360

B

Bisphosphonates
  complications of
    esophageal cancer, 394–395

Rheum Dis Clin N Am 37 (2011) 479–488
doi:10.1016/S0889-857X(11)00053-6
0889-857X/11/$ – see front matter © 2011 Elsevier Inc. All rights reserved.

Bisphosphonates (*continued*)
    fractures, 391–394
    osteonecrosis of jaw, 387–391
  discontinuation of, **323–336**
    bone mineral density effects of, 324–327
    bone turnover marker effects of, 324–327
    decisions concerning, 329–332
    fracture risk after, 327–332
  drug holiday for, 331, 396
  for glucocorticoid-induced osteoporosis, 419–420
  for men, 407
  mechanism of action of, 339
  risks versus benefits of, 395–396
  switching to teriparatide from, 331
  teriparatide after, 474
Bone mineral density
  for fracture prediction, 366
  glucocorticoid effects on, 417–418
  in men, 403–405
  treatment discontinuation effects on, 324–327
Bone remodeling, physiology of, 337–338
Bone turnover markers, **365–386**
  assays for, 370–371
  characteristics of, 367–368
  diagnostic use of, 368
  for complication prevention, 381
  for fracture risk assessment, 369, 373
  for prediction of bone loss, 373–374
  for therapeutic response prediction, 375–381
  for therapy choice, 374–375
  persistence of therapy and, 381
  physiology of, 365–367
  treatment discontinuation effects on, 324–327
Bone-specific alkaline phosphatase (BSAP). *See* BSAP (bone-specific alkaline
  phosphatase).
Breast cancer
  aromatase inhibitors for, denosumab with, 447–448
  vitamin D and, 357–358
BSAP (bone-specific alkaline phosphatase)
  assays for, 372
  denosumab effects on, 438–439
  diagnostic use of, 368
  for fracture risk assessment, 369
  for prediction of bone loss, 373–374
  for therapeutic response prediction, 375, 379–380
  for therapy choice, 374–375

C

Calcitonin, 422
Calcium

cardiovascular risk with, 356–357
dosing of, 351–356
for men, 407
recommendations for, 360
toxicity of, 353–354
with glucocorticoid therapy, 418
Calcium-sensing receptor, 346–347
Canadian Multicenter Osteoporosis Study (CaMOS), 342
Cancer
esophageal, bisphosphonate-induced, 394–395
vitamin D and, 357–358
Carboxy-terminal crosslinking telopeptide of type I collagen generated by
matrixmetalloproteinases (CTP), assays for, 370
Cardiovascular disease, vitamin D and calcium supplementation and, 356–357
Cathepsin K inhibitors, 339–341
Colon cancer, vitamin D and, 358
Continuing Outcomes Relevant to Evista (CORE), 328
CORE (Continuing Outcomes Relevant to Evista), 328
Coronary artery disease, vitamin D and calcium supplementation and, 356–357
Corticosteroids. See Glucocorticoid-induced osteoporosis.
CTP (carboxy-terminal crosslinking telopeptide of type I collagen generated by
matrixmetalloproteinases), assays for, 370
CTX (carboxy-terminal crosslinking telopeptide of type 1 collagen)
assays for, 370
denosumab effects on, 435–445
diagnostic use of, 368
for fracture risk assessment, 369, 373
for prediction of bone loss, 373–374
for therapeutic response prediction, 375, 379–380
for therapy choice, 374–375
CTX-MMP (carboxy-terminal crosslinking telopeptide of type I collagen generated by
matrixmetalloproteinases), assays for, 370
Cyclic teriparatide, 475

D

DAPS (Denosumab Adherence Preference Satisfaction Study), 446–447
DECIDE (Determining Efficacy: Comparison of Initiating Denosumab vs. Alendronate)
trial, 445–446
DEFEND (Denosumab Fortifies Bone Density) trial, 440–442
Denosumab, 433–452
adverse events with, 439–442
clinical studies of, 436–440
aromatase inhibitors with, 447–448
fracture prevention, 442–444
men with androgen deprivation therapy, 447
patient satisfaction, 446–447
postmenopausal women, 436–442, 445–446
single-dose, dose-escalation study of, 435–436
transitioning from alendronate, 445
discontinuation of

Denosumab (*continued*)
    bone mineral density effects of, 326
    bone turnover marker effects of, 326
    fracture risk after, 329
  response to, bone turnover markers for, 378
  versus alendronate, 445–447
Denosumab Adherence Preference Satisfaction Study (DAPS), 446–447
Denosumab Fortifies Bone Density (DEFEND) trial, 440–442
Dental Practice-Based Research Network, 390
Deoxypyridinoline (DPD)
  assays for, 371
  for therapy choice, 374
Department of Veterans Affairs, osteoporosis screening guidelines of, 404–405
Determining Efficacy: Comparison of Initiating Denosumab vs. Alendronate
  (DECIDE) trial, 445–446
Diabetes mellitus
  bone turnover markers in, 373
  vitamin D and, 359
Dialysis, teriparatide for, 476
Diaphyseal fractures, bisphosphonate-induced, 391–394
Dickkopf-1, 342–345
DPD (deoxypyridinoline)
  assays for, 371
  for therapy choice, 374
Drug holiday, 331, 396
Dual-energy X-ray absorptiometry, 366

E

EPIDOS study, 369
Esophageal cancer, bisphosphonate-induced, 394–395
Estrogen(s), 422
  discontinuation of
    bone mineral density effects of, 326
    bone turnover marker effects of, 325–326
    fracture risk after, 328
  selection of, bone turnover markers for, 374
Etidronate, for glucocorticoid-induced osteoporosis, 419–420
European Study of Forsteo (EUROFORS), 474

F

Femoral fractures
  bisphosphonate-induced, 391–394
  teriparatide effects on, 476
FIT (Fracture Intervention Trial), 374
FLEX (Fracture Intervention Trial Long Term Extension), 325, 328
Fracture(s)
  diaphyseal, bisphosphonate-induced, 391–394
  healing of, teriparatide effects on, 475–476
  in men, 402–403

risk of
    after treatment discontinuation, 327–332
    bone turnover markers and, 369, 373
    in glucocorticoid therapy, 417–418
    subtrochanteric, bisphosphonate-induced, 391–394, 476
Fracture Intervention Trial (FIT), 374
Fracture Intervention Trial Long Term Extension (FLEX), 325, 328
Fracture Prevention Trial (FPT), 328, 374
Fracture Reduction evaluation of Denosumab in Osteoporosis Every 6 Months
    (FREEDOM) trial, 380, 442–444
Fracture Risk Assessment Tool (FRAX), 366–367, 369, 401–402, **453–471**
    adjustments to, 465–467
    Canadian, 457–458
    caveats for, 459–460
    clinical risk factors in, 454–458, 460–461
    clinician's guide for, 461–462
    demographics in, 456
    development of, 454–455
    Implementation Guide for, 458–459
    limitations of, 461–462
    official positions for, 463–465
    Position Development Conference for, 463–465
    strengths of, 461–462
FRAX. See Fracture Risk Assessment Tool (FRAX).
FREEDOM trial, 380, 442–444
FTP (Fracture Prevention Trial), 328

G

Garvan Institute fracture risk calculator, 454, 461
General Practice Research Database, 327
Glucagonlike peptide 2, 341–32
Glucocorticoid-induced osteoporosis, **415–437**
    bone mineral density in, 417
    fracture risk in, 417–418
    in men, 408
    pathogenesis of, 415–416
    treatment of
        bisphosphonates for, 419–420
        nonpharmacologic, 418–419
        recommendations for, 422–427
        teriparatide for, 420–422, 476–477

H

Health Outcomes and Reduced Incidence with Zolendronic Acid Once Yearly Pivotal
    Fracture Trial (HORIZON PFT), 326, 328
Hip, transient osteoporosis of, 476
Hip fractures
    bisphosphonate-induced, 391–394
    in men, 402–403

Hip (*continued*)
    teriparatide effects on, 476
HORIZON PFT (Health Outcomes and Reduced Incidence with Zolendronic
    Acid Once Yearly Pivotal Fracture Trial), 326, 328
HORIZON-GIOP, 420
Hormone therapy, 422
    discontinuation of
        bone mineral density effects of, 326
        bone turnover marker effects of, 325–326
        fracture risk after, 328
Hydroxyproline (HYP), assays for, 371
Hyperparathyroidism, in vitamin D deficiency, 352–353
Hypogonadism, 405–406, 416

I

Ibandronate
    discontinuation of
        bone mineral density effects of, 325
        bone turnover marker effects of, 325
    for glucocorticoid-induced osteoporosis, 420
    response to, bone turnover markers for, 378
    selection of, bone turnover markers for, 375
Inflammatory bowel disease, vitamin D and, 359–360
International Osteoporosis Foundation, 366, 457, 464
International Society of Clinical Densitometry, position statement on testing for men, 404

J

Jaw, osteonecrosis of, 387–391, 476

K

Kidney failure, teriparatide for, 476

M

Macrophage colony-stimulating factor, 416
Mandible, osteonecrosis of, 387–391, 476
Manitoba Bone Density Program, 457
Maxilla, osteonecrosis of, 387–391, 476
Men, osteoporosis in, **401–414**
    bone turnover markers in, 369
    denosumab for, 447
    diagnosis of, 404–406
    epidemiology of, 401–403
    risk factors for, 403–404
    treatment of, 407–408
Multiple Outcomes of Raloxifene Evaluation (MORE), 328
Multiple sclerosis, vitamin D and, 359–360
Myocardial infarction, vitamin D and calcium supplementation and, 356–357

N

National Osteoporosis Foundation
   FRAX validation by, 457–459
   on epidemiology, 402
Nitrates, 342
Nitroglycerine as an Option: Value in Early Bone Loss (NOVEL) trial, 342
Nordic Research on Ageing (NORA) study, 367
NOVEL (Nitroglycerine as an Option: Value in Early Bone Loss) trial, 342
NTX (amino-terminal crosslinking telopeptide of type I collagen)
   assays for, 370
   denosumab effects on, 435–439
   diagnostic use of, 368
   for prediction of bone loss, 373–374
   for therapeutic response prediction, 375, 379
   for therapy choice, 374

O

OC. *See* Osteocalcin (OC).
Odanacatib, 339–341
OFELY study, 369
Osteoblasts, function of, 337–338
Osteocalcin (OC)
   assays for, 372
   diagnostic use of, 368
   for prediction of bone loss, 373–374
   for therapeutic response prediction, 375
   for therapy choice, 374
Osteoclasts, function of, 337–338
Osteocytes, function of, 337–338
Osteonecrosis, of jaw, 387–391, 476
Osteopenia, definition of, 369
Osteoporosis
   assessment of
      bone turnover markers for, **365–386**
      for fracture risk, **453–471**
      teriparatide in, **473–479**
   diagnosis of
      bone turnover markers for, 368
      in men, 404–406
   epidemiology of, in men, 401–403
   glucocorticoid-induced, 408, **415–437**
   in men, **404–414**
   RANKL pathway in, **433–452**
   risk factors for, in men, 403–404
   secondary, 405–407
   treatment of
      calcium and vitamin D for, **351–365**
      denosumab for, **433–452**
      duration of, **323–336**

Osteoporosis (*continued*)
    emerging, **337–350**
    evaluation of, bone turnover markers for, **365–386**
    in men, 407–408
    safety of, **387–400**
Osteoporosis pseudoglioma, 344–345
Osteoprotegerin, 373, 434

P

Pain, in osteoporosis, teriparatide for, 476
Pamidronate
    for glucocorticoid-induced osteoporosis, 419–420
    selection of, bone turnover markers for, 374
Parathyroid hormone
    calcium-sensing receptor and, 346–347
    for therapy. *See* Teriparatide.
    replacement of, 347–348
    response to, bone turnover markers for, 379–380
Parathyroid Hormone and Alendronate for Osteoporosis trial, 473–474
Parathyroid-related protein, 347–348
PICP (procollagen type I carboxy-terminal propeptide)
    assays for, 372
    for therapeutic response prediction, 375–376, 379
    for therapy choice, 374–375
PINP (procollagen type I amino-terminal propeptide)
    assays for, 372
    for therapeutic response prediction, 375–376, 380
    for therapy choice, 374–375
Prednisone
    fracture risk from, 460–461, 466
    osteoporosis prevention with, 418–419
Procollagen type I amino-terminal propeptide. *See* PINP (procollagen type I amino-terminal propeptide).
Procollagen type I carboxy-terminal propeptide. *See* PICP (procollagen type I carboxy-terminal propeptide).
Pseudoglioma, osteoporosis, 344–345
Pycnodysostosis, 339
Pyridinoline (PYD), assays for, 371

Q

QFractureScores, 454, 461

R

Raloxifene
    discontinuation of
        bone mineral density effects of, 326
        bone turnover marker effects of, 325–326
        fracture risk after, 329

response to, bone turnover markers for, 378, 380
RANK and RANKL pathway, 416, **433–452**
    action of, 434
    denosumab and, **433–452**
    treatment implications of, 434–435
Receptor activator of nuclear factor κB (RANK). See RANK and RANKL pathway.
Rheumatoid arthritis, vitamin D and, 359
Risedronate
    discontinuation of
        bone mineral density effects of, 325
        bone turnover marker effects of, 325
        fracture risk after, 328–332
    for glucocorticoid-induced osteoporosis, 419–420
    for men, 407
    response to, bone turnover markers for, 378
    selection of, bone turnover markers for, 374–375
Ronacaleret (SB-751689), 347

S

Sclerosteosis, 343–344
Sclerostin, 342–345
Serotonin, 345–346
SOF (Study of Osteoporotic Fractures), 342, 454
STAND trial, 445
Strontium ranelate, 378–380
Study of Osteoporotic Fractures (SOF), 342, 454
Subtrochanteric fractures
    atypical, bisphosphonate-induced, 391–394, 476
    teriparatide effects on, 476
Systemic lupus erythematosus, vitamin D and, 359

T

Tartrate-resistant acid phosphatase (TRACP), assays for, 371
Teriparatide
    adherence to, 477
    after bisphosphonates, 474
    cyclic, 475
    discontinuation of
        bone mineral density effects of, 326–327
        bone turnover marker effects of, 326–327
        fracture risk after, 329
    follow-up for, 474–475
    for glucocorticoid-induced osteoporosis, 420–422, 476–477
    for kidney disease, 476
    for men, 407
    for osteonecrosis of jaw, 476
    for pain management, 476
    fracture healing with, 475–476
    response to, bone turnover markers for, 375–379

Teriparatide (*continued*)
    switching from bisphosphonates to, 331
    zolendronate with, 473–474
Testosterone
    for men, 407–408
    low levels of, 406–407
TRACP (tartrate-resistant acid phosphatase), assays for, 371
Transient osteoporosis, of hip, 476
T-score, in FRAX, 467

U

United Kingdom General Proteic Database study, of glucocorticoid-induced
    osteoporosis, 417

V

Vertebral Efficacy with Risedronate Therapy-North American (VERT-NA) trial, 325, 328
Vitamin D
    autoimmune disease development and, 358–360
    cancer development and, 357–358
    cardiovascular risk with, 356–357
    dosing of, 351–356
    for men, 407
    recommendations for, 360
    screening for, 360
    toxicity of, 353–354
    with glucocorticoid therapy, 418

W

Wnt signaling, 342–345
Women's Health Initiative studies
    calcium with vitamin D supplementation, 357
    estrogen therapy, 327
World Health Organization
    osteoporosis definition of, 453
    osteoporosis intervention recommendations of, 366

Z

Zolendronate
    discontinuation of
        bone mineral density effects of, 325–326
        bone turnover marker effects of, 325–326
        fracture risk after, 328–332
    for glucocorticoid-induced osteoporosis, 420
    for men, 407
    response to, bone turnover markers for, 378, 380
    teriparatide with, 473–474